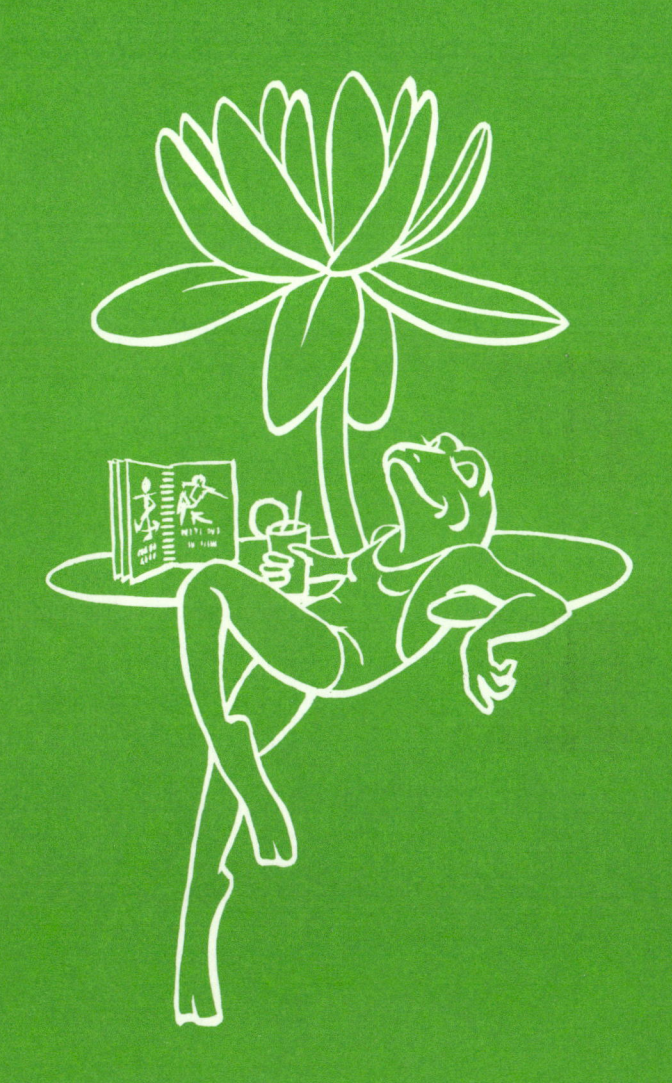

SHAPE-UP WITH *Splash*

WRITTEN BY
JUDY DAVENPORT CONLEY

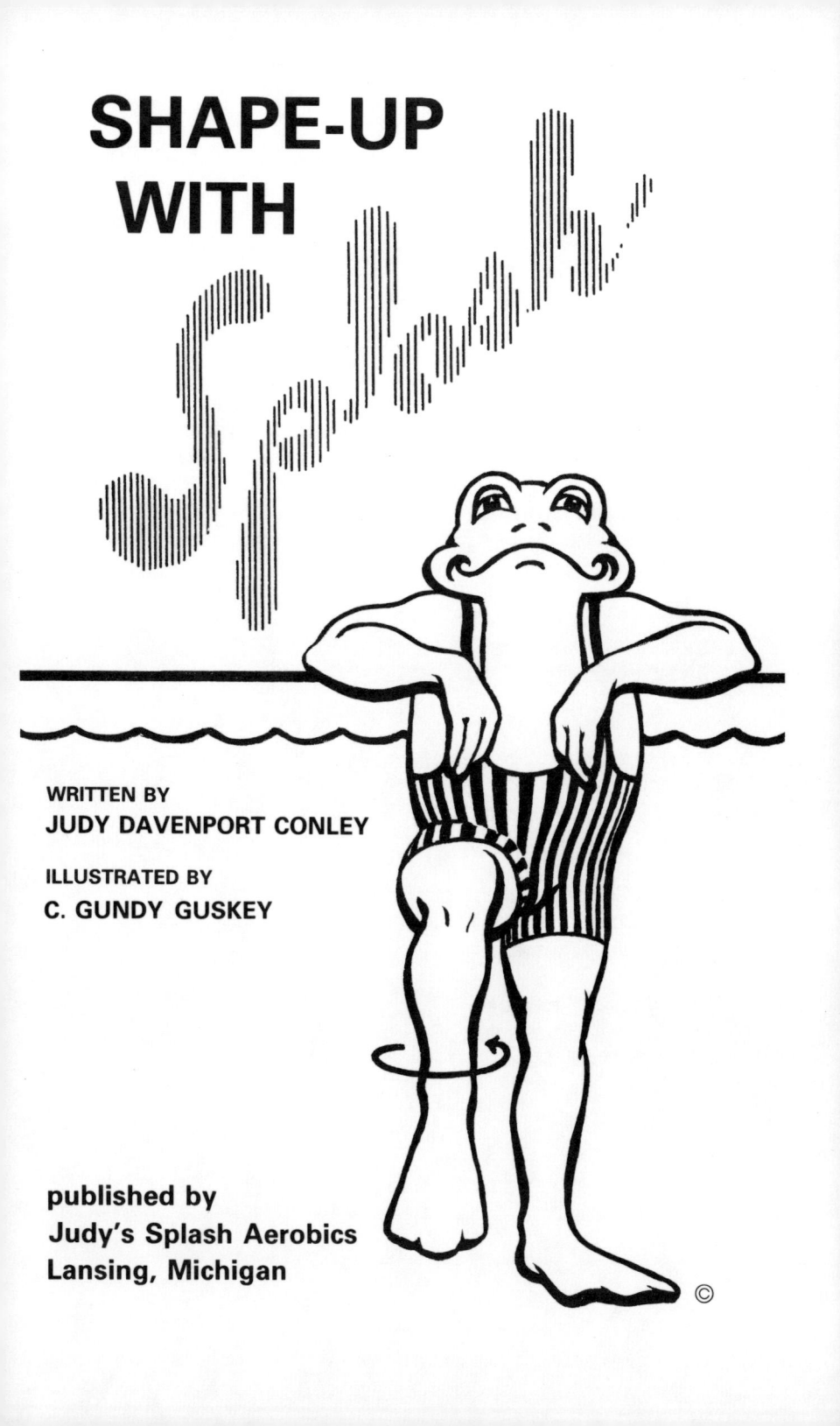

ILLUSTRATED BY
C. GUNDY GUSKEY

published by
Judy's Splash Aerobics
Lansing, Michigan

Copyright © 1988 by Judy's Splash Aerobics

All rights reserved. No part of this book may be reproduced or utilized in any form or by any means including but not limited to electronic or mechanical, including photocopying, recording, or by information storage or retrieval system, except for excerpts by health and exercise editors and magazines with proper credit, without permission in writing from the publisher.

Inquiries should be sent to:
Judy's Splash Aerobics
1738 Briarwood
Lansing, Michigan 48917

Printed in the United States of America
First printing April 1988
Second Printing August 1989
10 9 8 7 6 5 4 3 2

Library of Congress Cataloging in Publication Data
Conley, Judy Davenport 1942 –
Shape-up with Splash

    1. Aquatic exercises
Shape-up with Splash
ISBN 0-9619828-1-0

ACKNOWLEDGEMENTS

A very special thank you to:

My husband Chuck, our children Carol, Tom, Rob, Kathleen, Liz, Charles, David and Billy, for all of their input, cooperation and encouragement.

Carol Guskey, a very talented artist and good friend, for the hours she spent drawing "Splash". To her husband Lou and their children Fleur and L. J., for their contributions and for the months they shared their home with frogs.

Also thanks to all my students who have helped refine "jugging" techniques, willingly served as guinea pigs in experimental water exercises, and encouraged the various stages of this book.

ABOUT THIS BOOK

To All Swimmers and Non-Swimmers:

I've written this book for my students who like to winter in warmer climates and want to stay in shape by continuing their exercises in the water during the winter months.

This book is also geared for anyone who would like a simple, quick reference for stretching and firming water exercises.

After years of teaching various forms of exercise, my students and I discovered that by doing the same exercises in the water that we had done on land, we achieved quicker results. We had a refreshed energic feeling. Most of all, being in the water was fun.

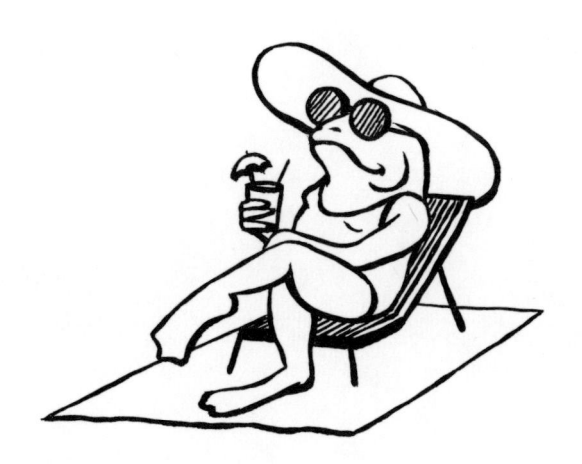

CONTENTS

HOW TO USE THIS BOOK	11
STRETCHING RULES	13
MY FAVORITE EXERCISES	25
WAIST AND ABDOMEN	27
SUPER TUMMY FLATTENER	41
THIGHS AND HIPS	47
ARMS	61
JUGGING RULES	77
JUGGING—ARMS	81
JUGGING—WAIST AND ABDOMEN	87
JUGGING—THIGHS AND HIPS	97
MY PROGRESS	103
CLEANSING CONTENTMENT	107

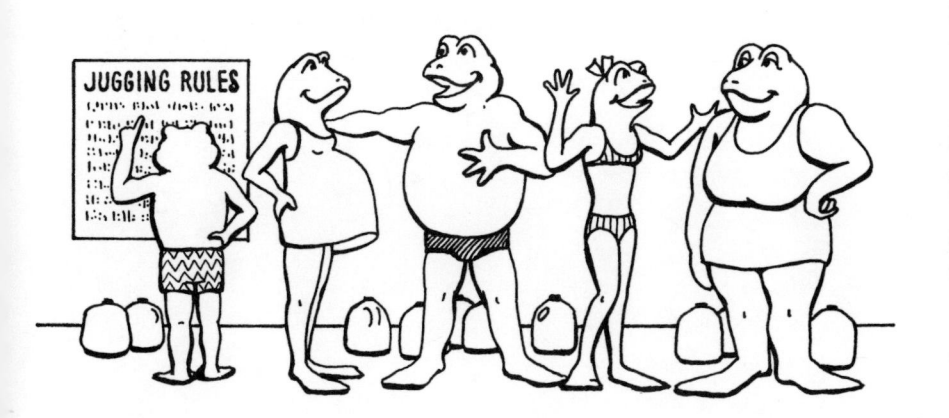

HOW TO USE THIS BOOK

If you've never exercised in the water, you're in for a special treat. Just pull in your stomach, tuck in your bottom, smile and enjoy a refreshing way to achieve a firmer more flexible body.

It is impossible to spot reduce but we can look better as our bodies become stronger and more flexible by working the various muscle groups.

So, put on a smile, hop into the water and lets get started:

Here are a few pointers:

1. Like any exercise program it is advisable to consult with your doctor before beginning. More doctors are becoming aware of the benefits of water programs.
2. Maintain good posture, tuck in your tummy, pull in your bottom and relax your shoulders and knees.
3. Think about the muscle that you're working and do the exercise correctly. The muscle being used is indicated by (\ ' /) in the illustrations.
4. If something hurts, don't do the exercise.
5. Select several exercises from each section. Start slowly and increase the intensity and number of exercises as you progress.
6. SMILE and ENJOY

STRETCHING RULES

1. Always warm up before stretching by walking around in the water swinging your arms
2. Always begin and end a work-out with at least 5 minutes of stretching
3. Avoid stress on a joint by never locking a joint
4. Hold a stretch at least 10–15 seconds — don't bounce a stretch
5. Repeat each stretch 3 or 4 times
6. Only stretch to the point that it "feels good"

SHOULDER ROLL

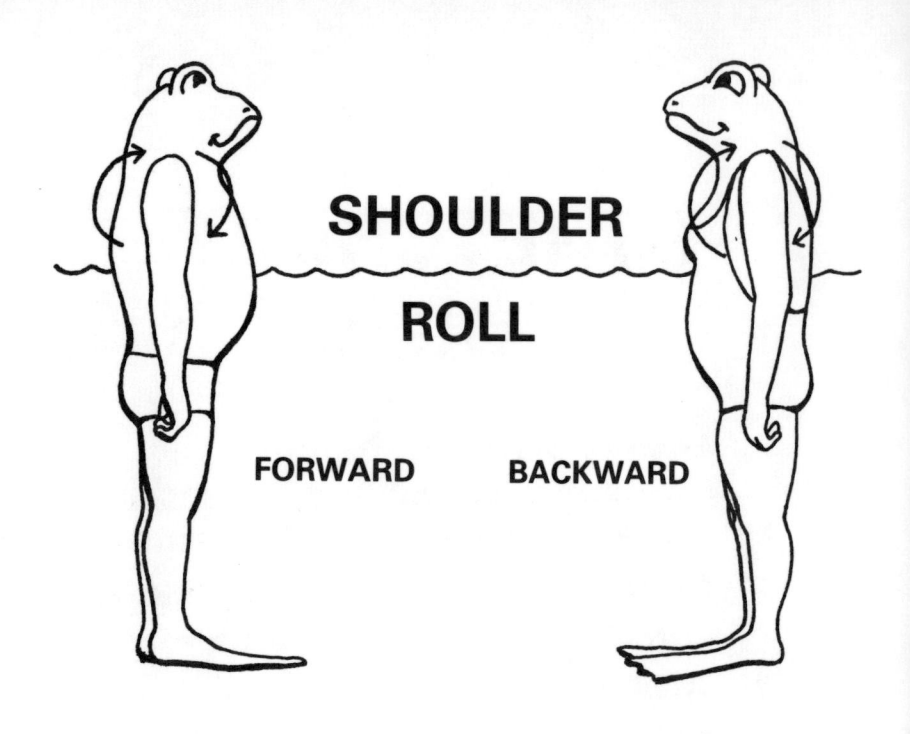

FORWARD   BACKWARD

HEAD ROLL

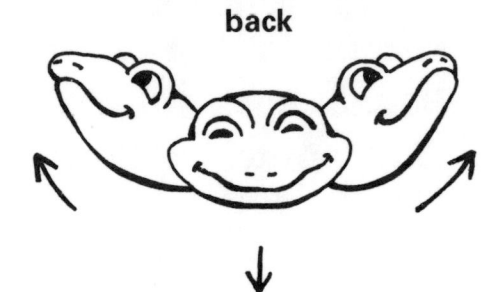

Don't roll head back

HEAD TURN

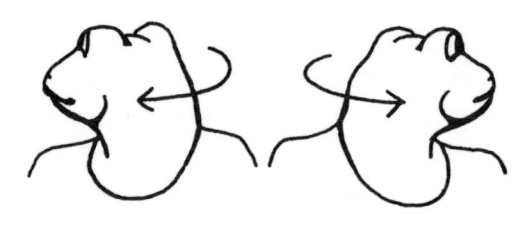

14 STRETCHING

TRUNK TWIST

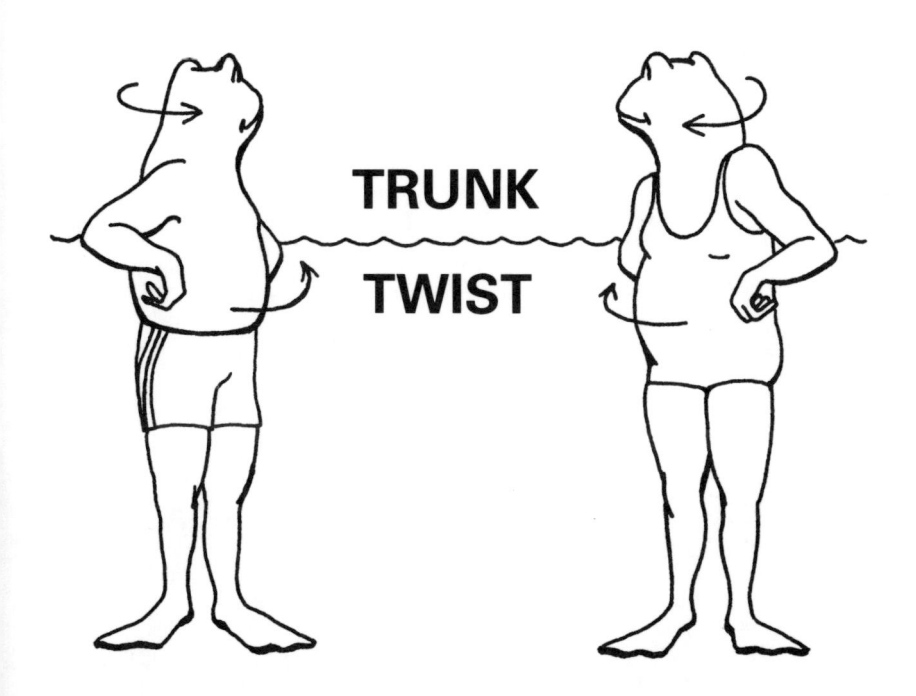

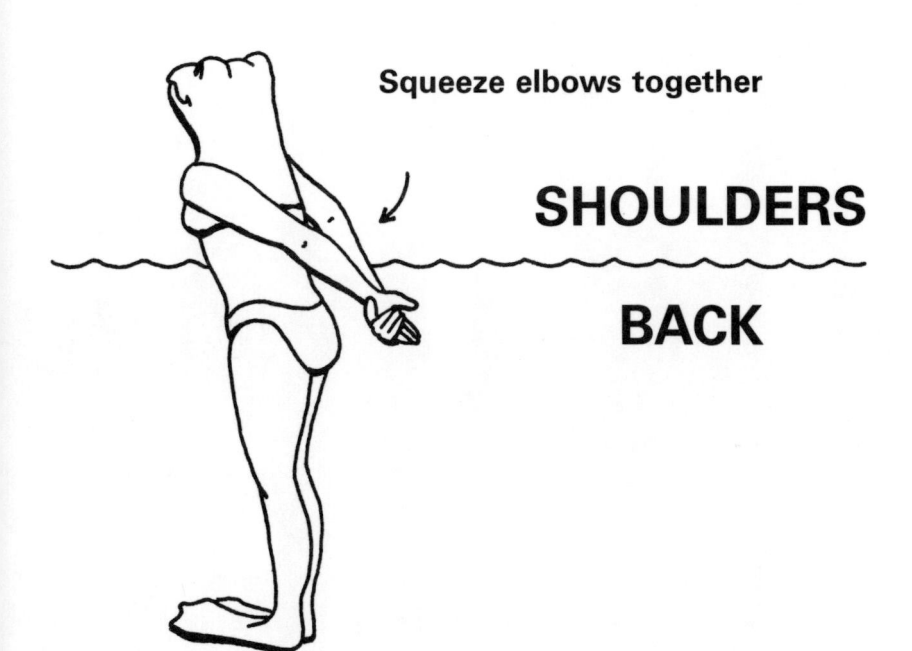

SHOULDERS BACK

Squeeze elbows together

SHOULDER STRETCH

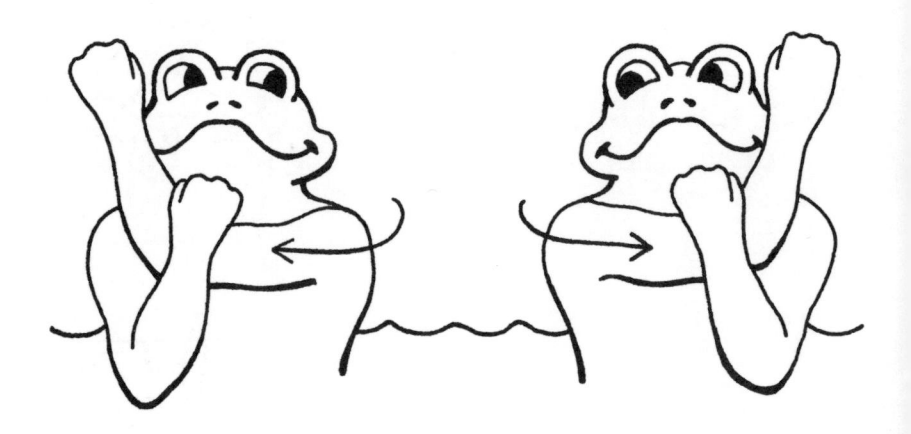

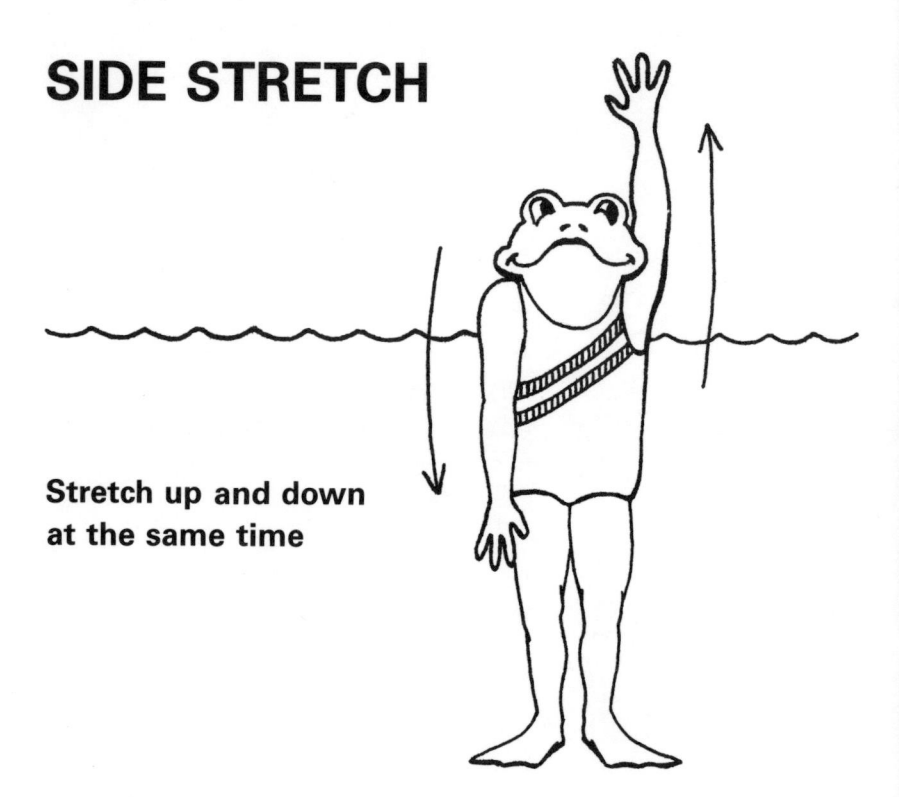

SIDE STRETCH

Stretch up and down at the same time

HIP STRETCH

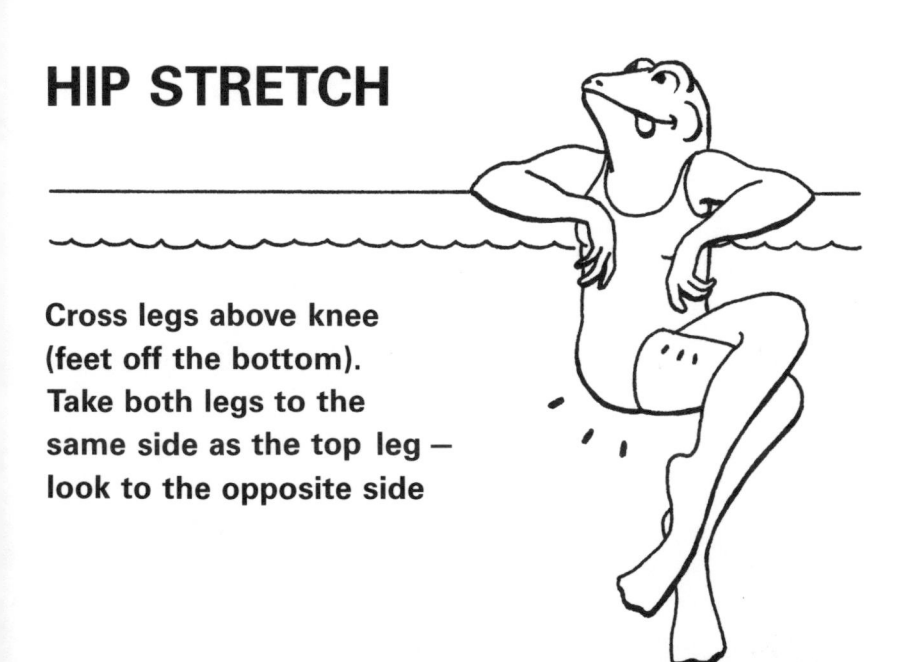

Cross legs above knee
(feet off the bottom).
Take both legs to the
same side as the top leg —
look to the opposite side

CALF/FOOT STRETCH
One foot on the wall with heel on the floor

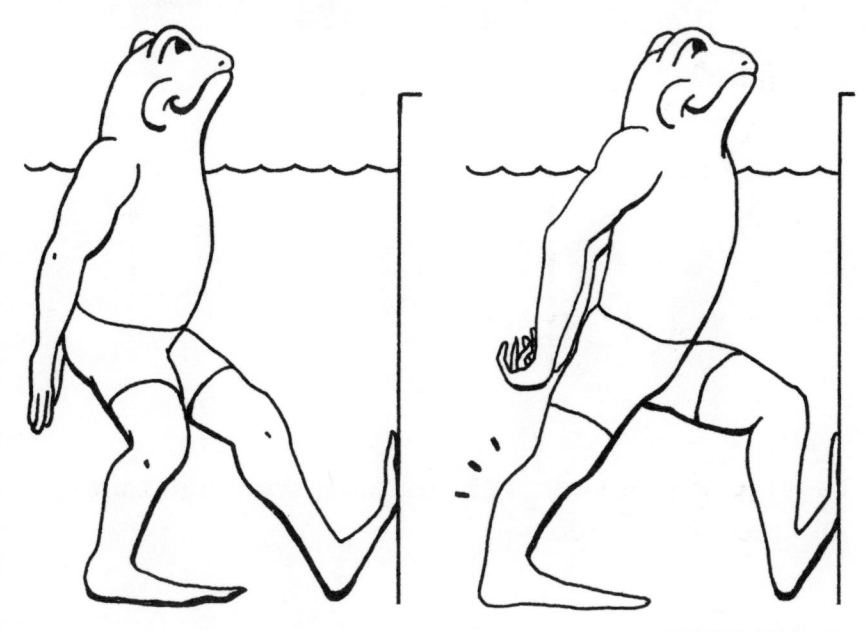

INNER THIGH STRETCH AGAINST WALL

TOP VIEW

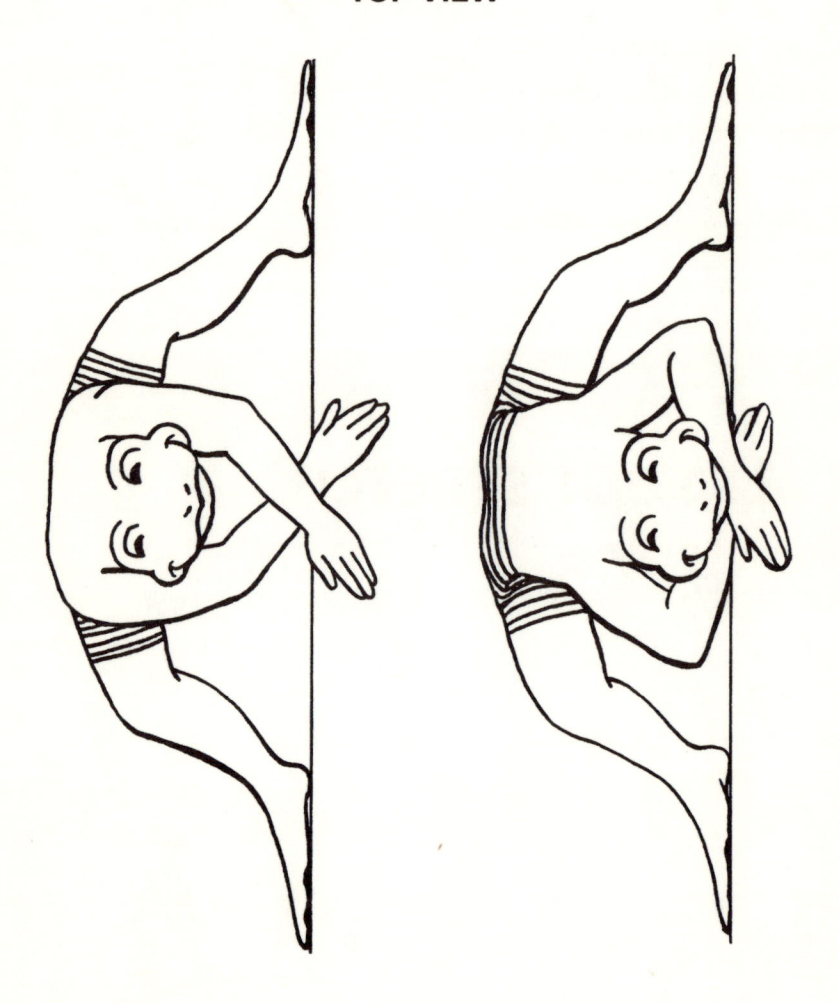

Legs high on the wall. Pull forward just enough to feel an inner thigh stretch

CALF STRETCH

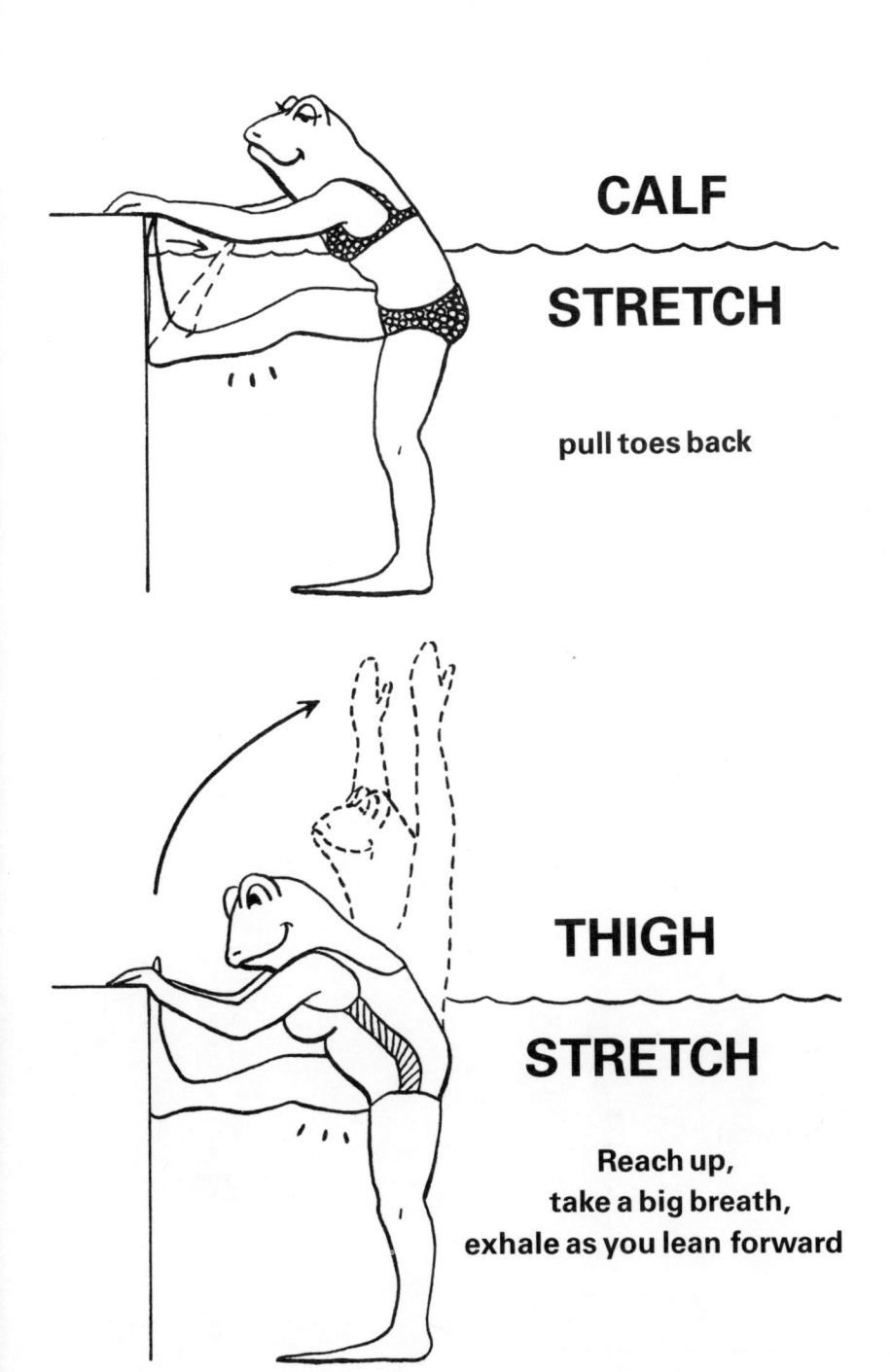

pull toes back

THIGH STRETCH

Reach up,
take a big breath,
exhale as you lean forward

THIGH STRETCH

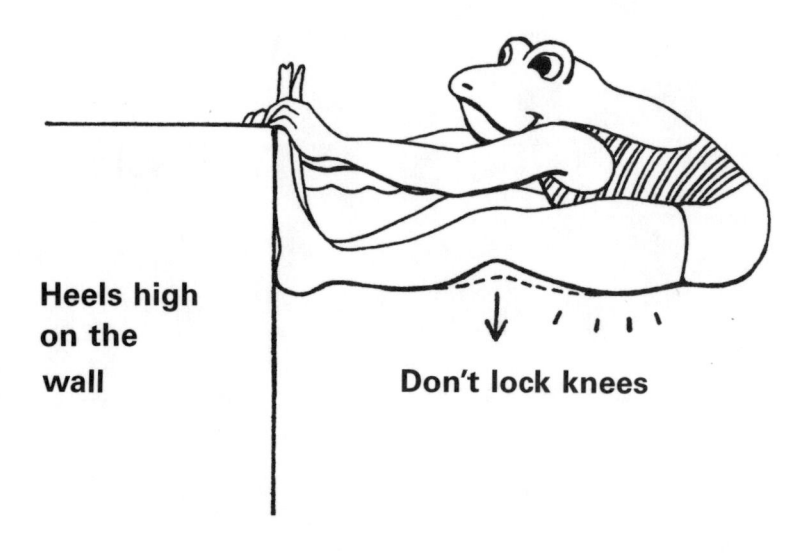

Heels high on the wall

Don't lock knees

CALF STRETCH

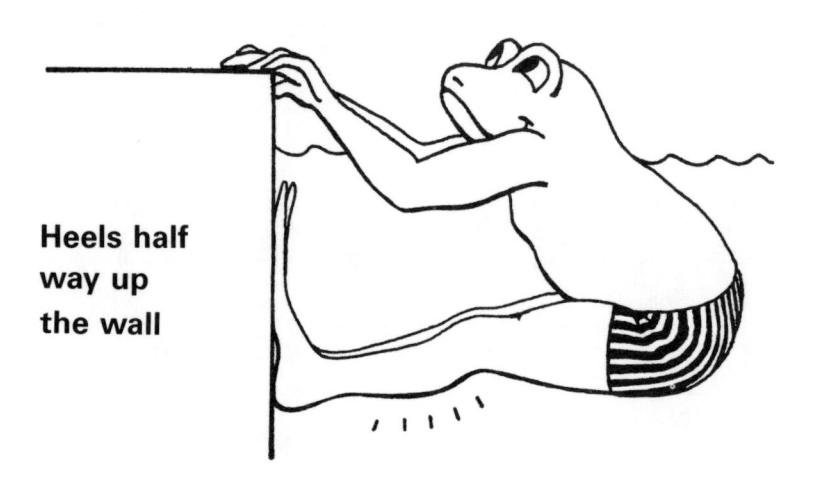

Heels half way up the wall

THIGH STRETCH

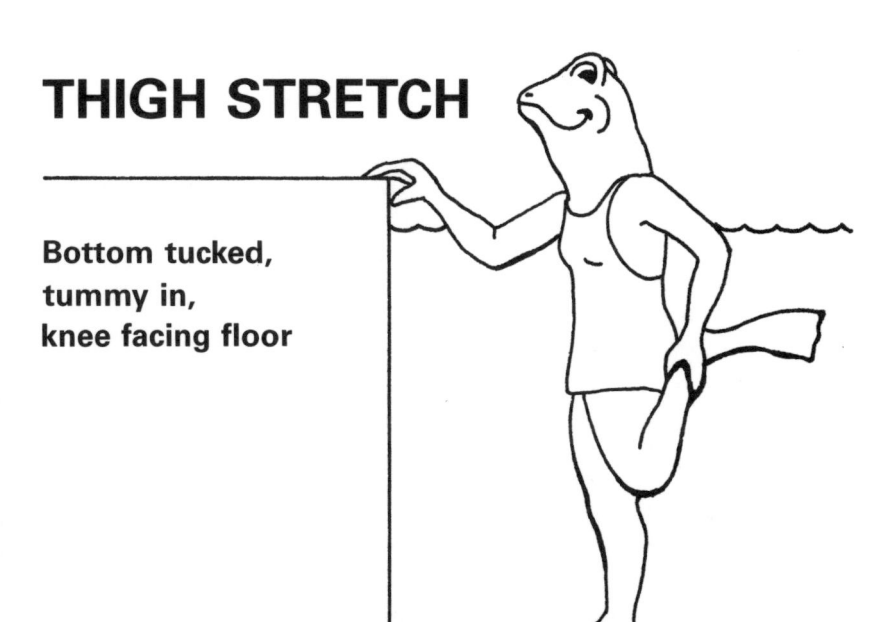

**Bottom tucked,
tummy in,
knee facing floor**

FOOT CRADLE

**Pull leg up close to body —
keep foot lower than knee**

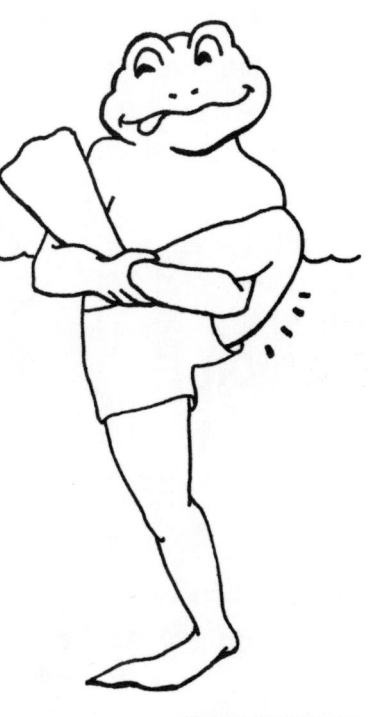

RUNNERS STRETCH
(inner thigh)

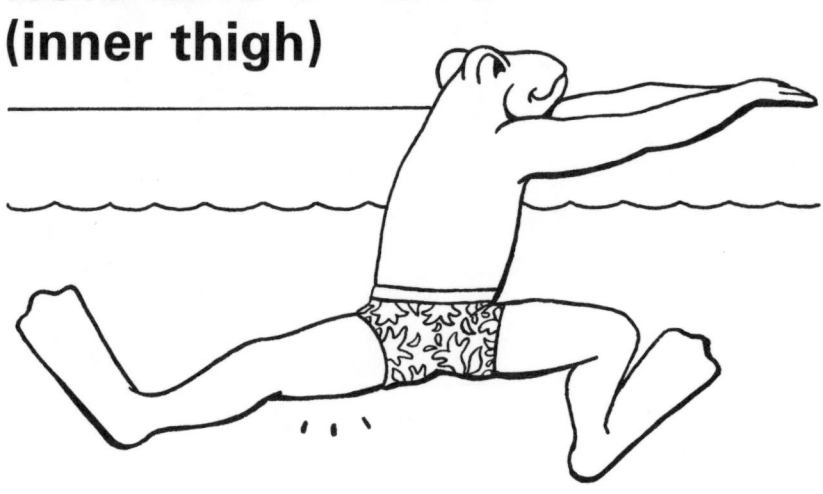

Begin with legs wide apart high on wall (holding onto pool edge or gutter with hands) Walk hands to side bending knee on that side — leave other leg straight (make sure knee faces toes not ceiling)

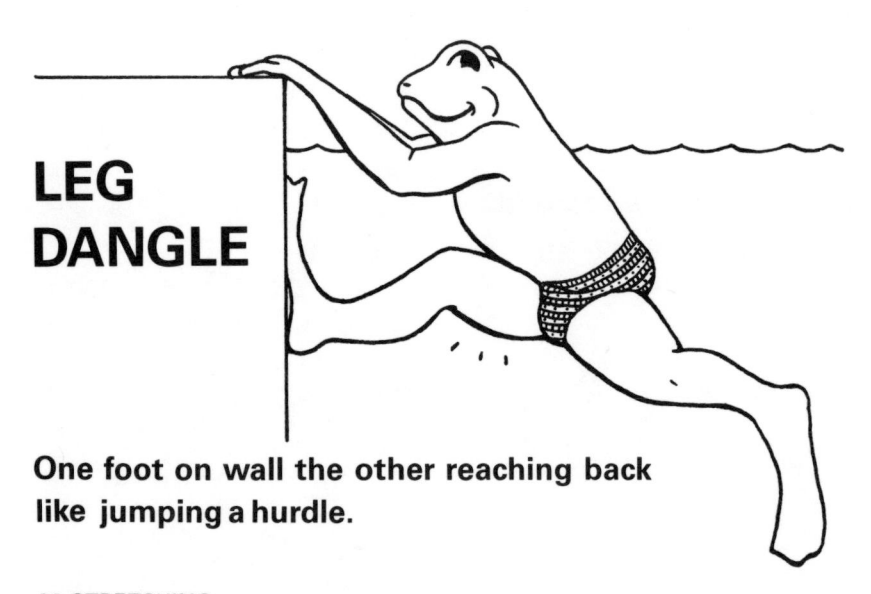

LEG DANGLE

One foot on wall the other reaching back like jumping a hurdle.

FOOT and ANKLE
(great relief from shoes that are too tight)

Holding leg up curl toes under, point foot, flex foot and release.

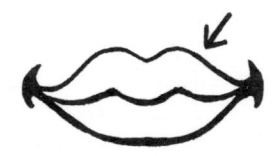

"REMEMBER" if you get a cramp pinch your upper lip...cramp should go away

FLAT BACK

Back to the wall — arch back
Then push one vertebrae at a time snug to the wall   Knees relaxed

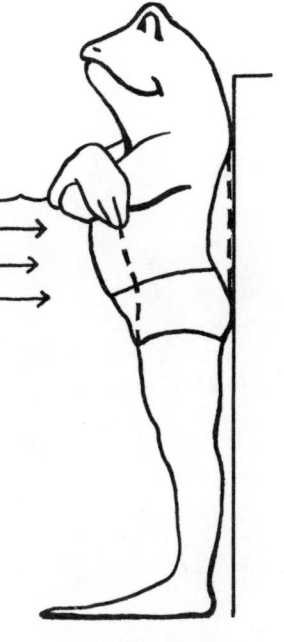

STRETCHING 23

GOOD
FEELING
STRETCH

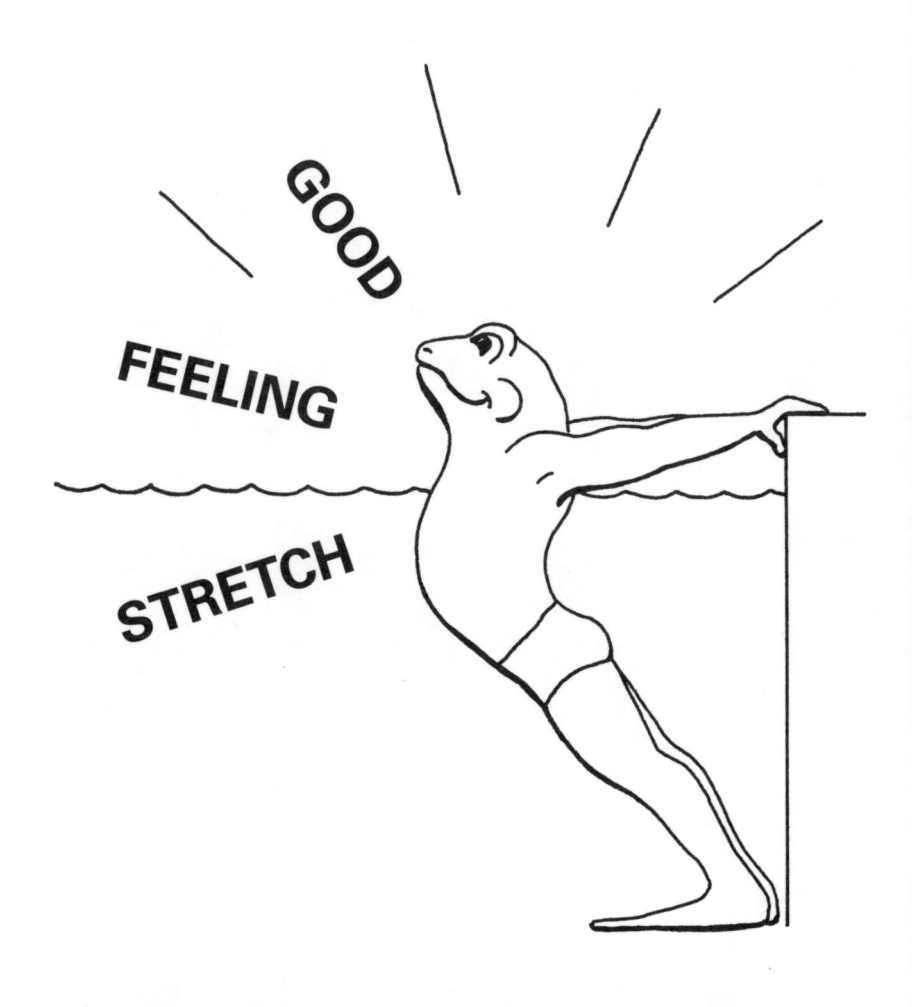

Back to wall, hands on gutter or pool edge —
Squeeze shoulder blades and elbows together,
stretching away from the wall — relax by
collapsing back into wall

MY FAVORITE EXERCISES

| STRETCHES | PAGE |

ARMS

WAIST AND ABDOMEN

THIGHS AND HIPS

JUGGING—ARMS

JUGGING—WAIST AND ABDOMEN

JUGGING—THIGHS AND HIPS

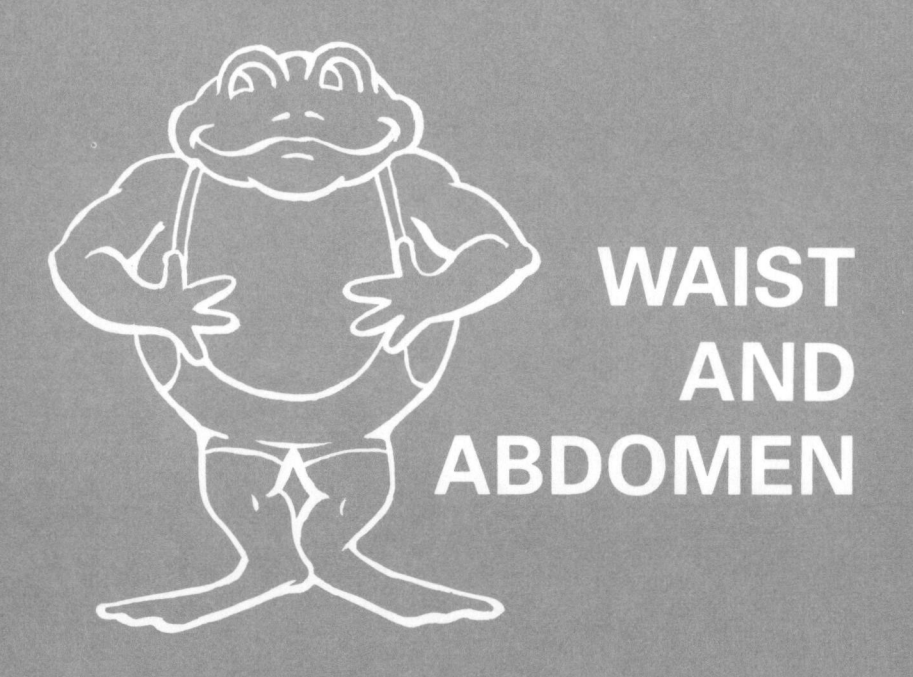

WAIST AND ABDOMEN

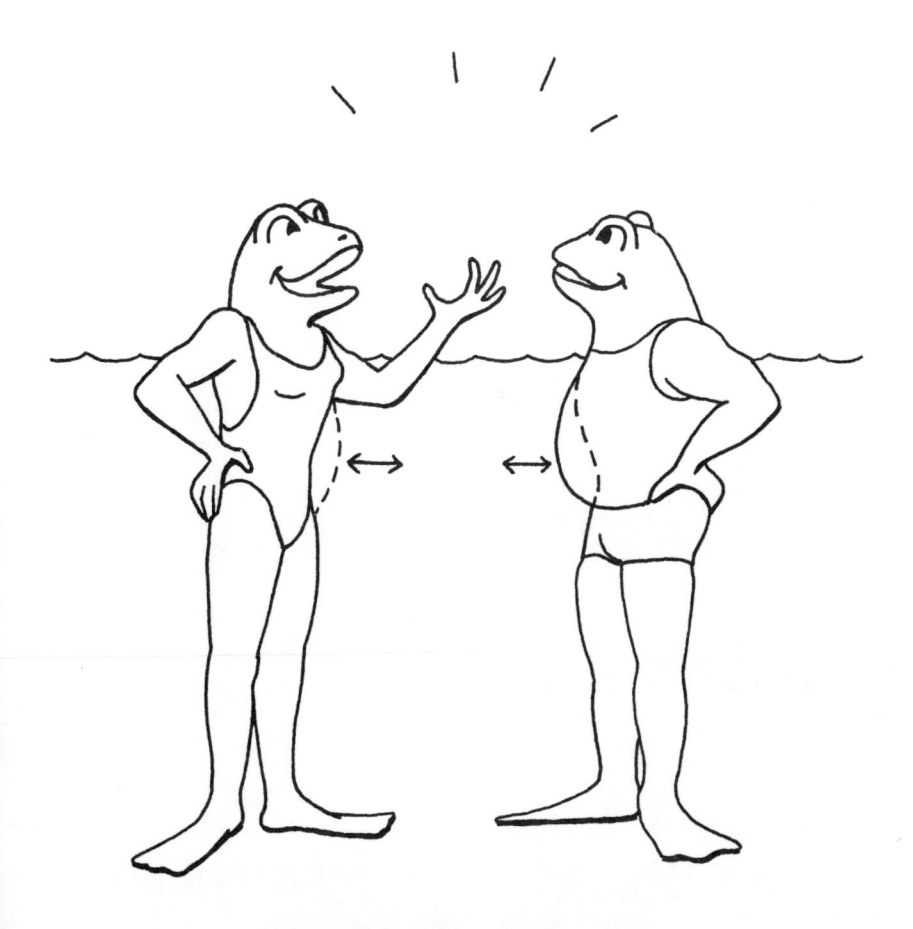

TUMMY CHATS

Talk and breathe normally while pushing stomach in and out

WAIST AND ABDOMEN 29

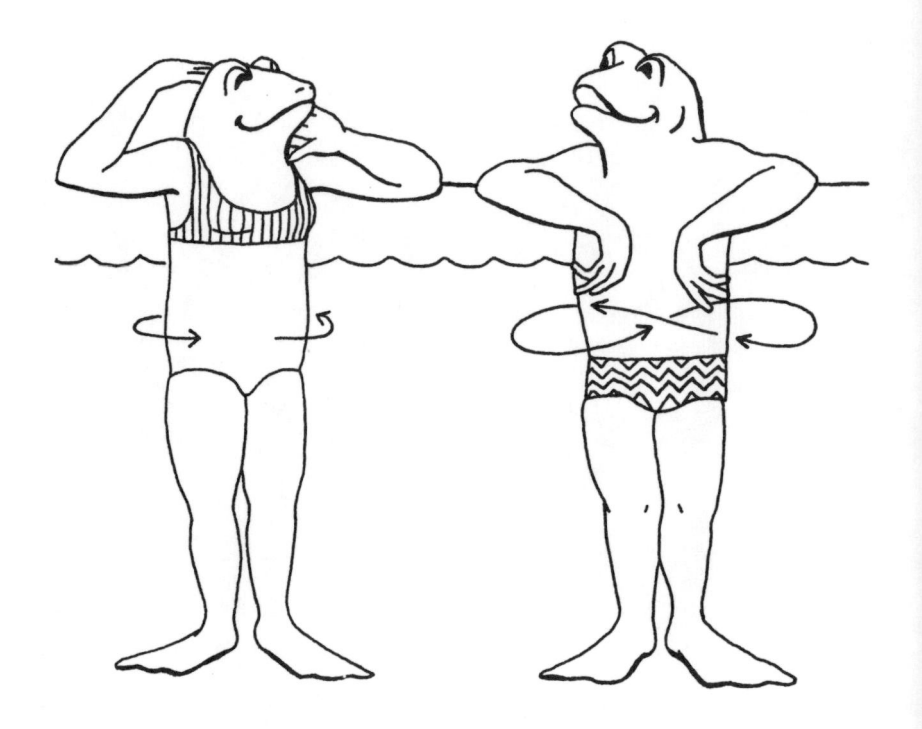

HULA HIP CIRCLES   FIGURE 8's

Keep knees relaxed — slightly bent

30 WAIST AND ABDOMEN

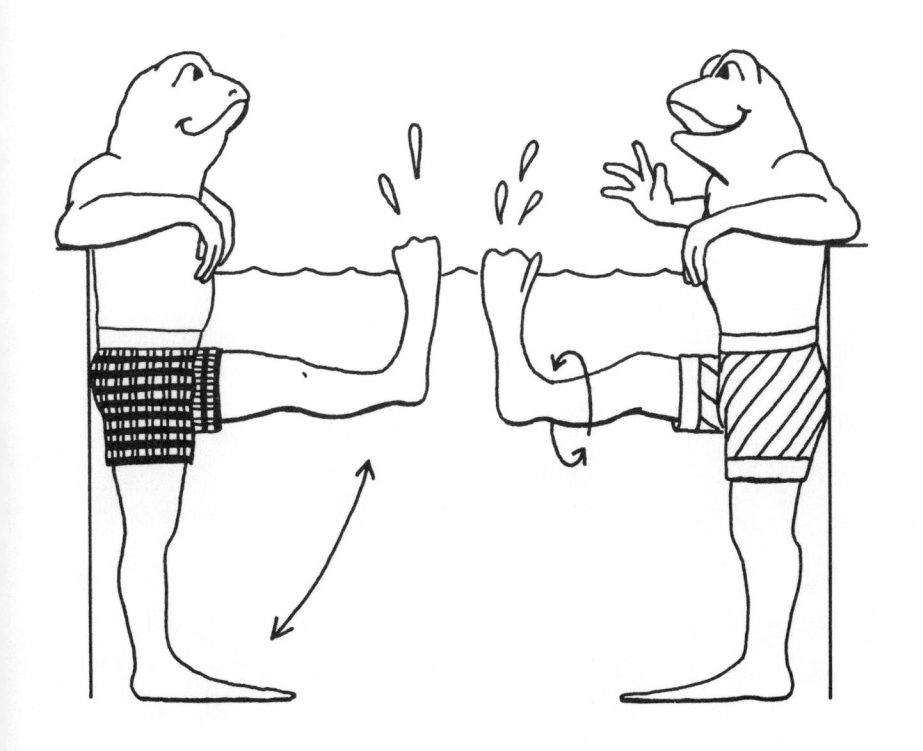

LEG LIFTS AND CIRCLES

Slowly raise leg and slowly take back to the floor
Slowly make small circles gradually getting larger then smaller

WAIST AND ABDOMEN

WIDE SWEEPS

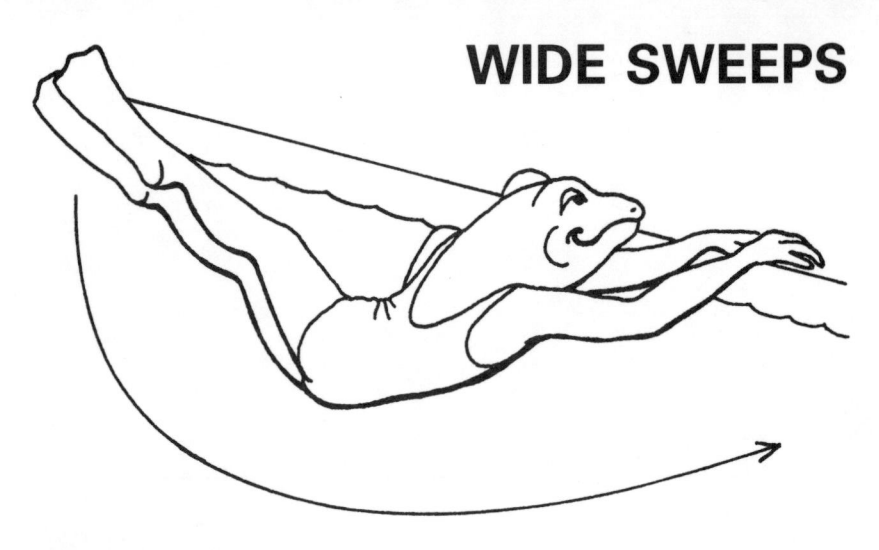

Keep body tight
Wide surface swing to the right and left — legs go straight out in back inbetween

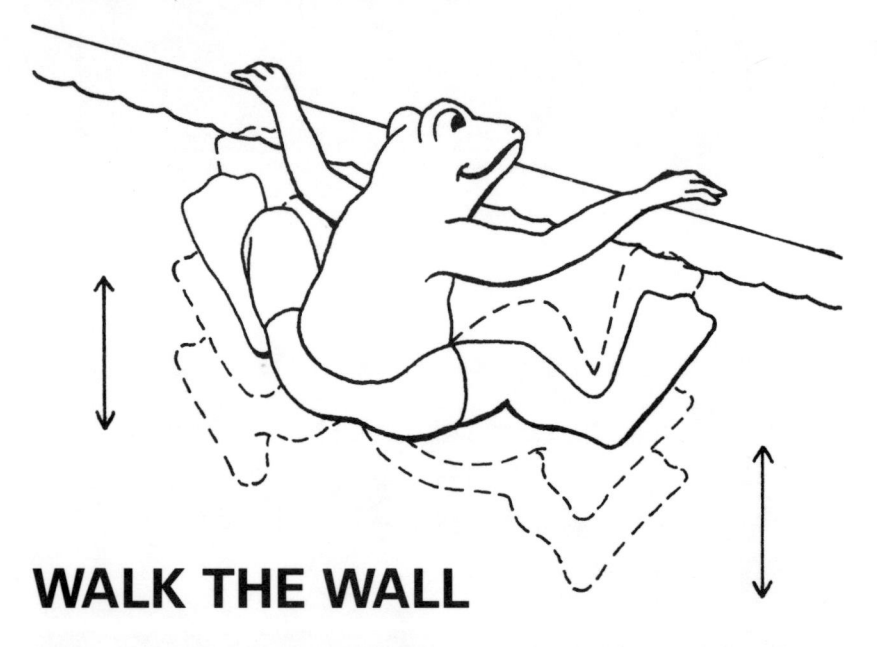

WALK THE WALL

Legs apart heels on the wall — walk up the wall and down (when heels come off the wall go the other direction)

32 WAIST AND ABDOMEN

FEET TOGETHER –

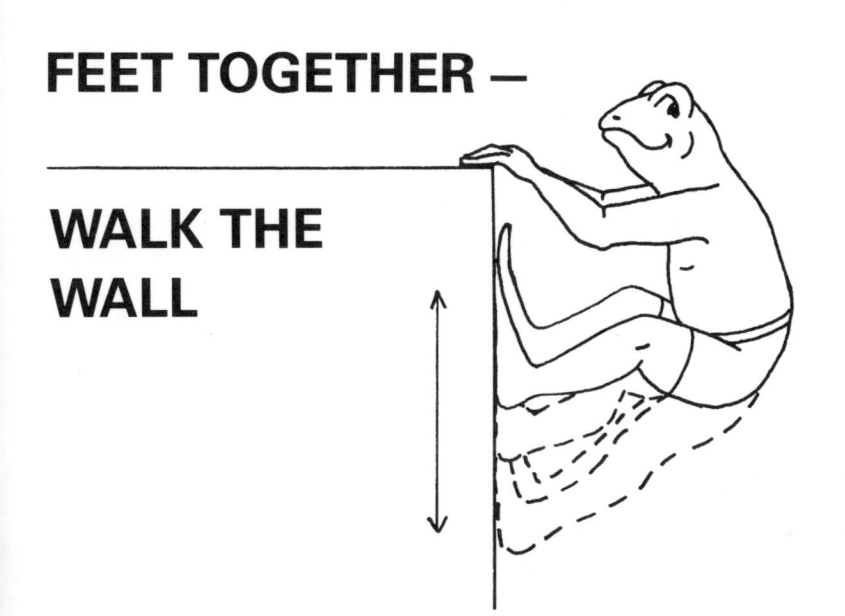

WALK THE WALL

WALKING TO EACH HAND

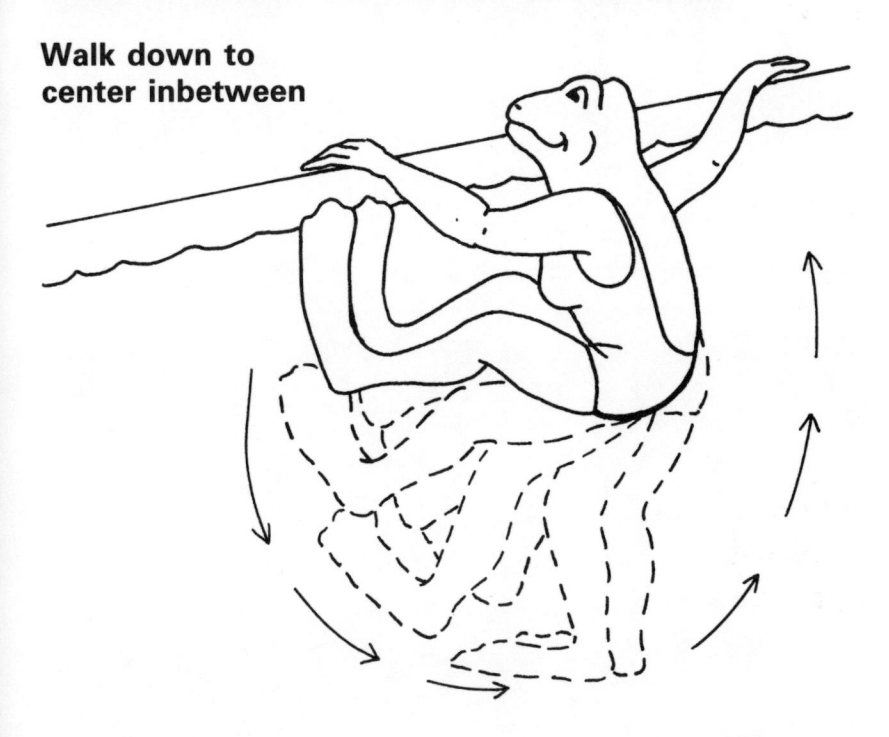

Walk down to center inbetween

WAIST AND ABDOMEN 33

"U" SWING

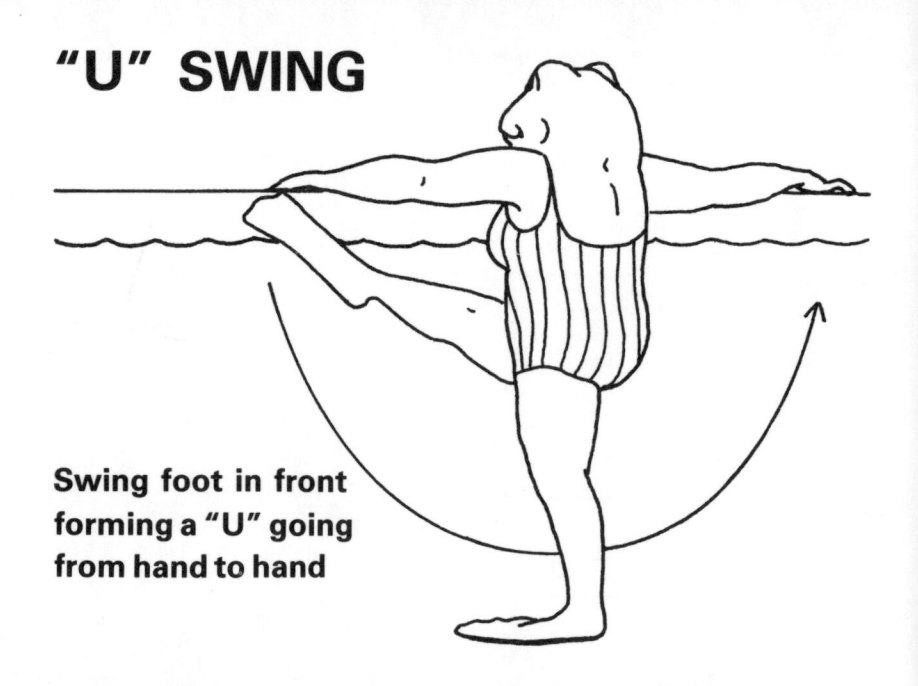

Swing foot in front forming a "U" going from hand to hand

MIDRIFF SLIMMER

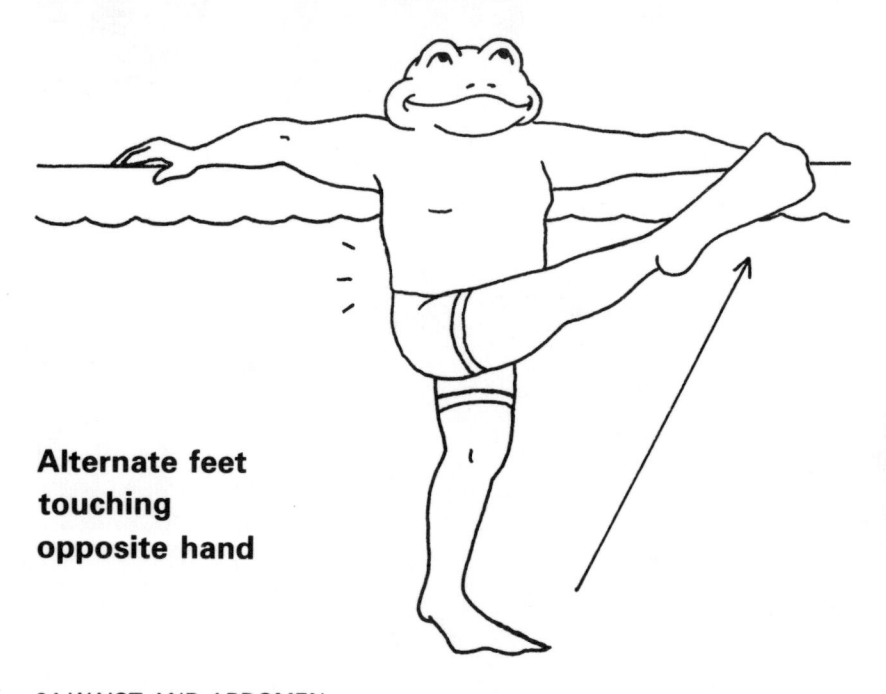

Alternate feet touching opposite hand

34 WAIST AND ABDOMEN

SIDE BENDS

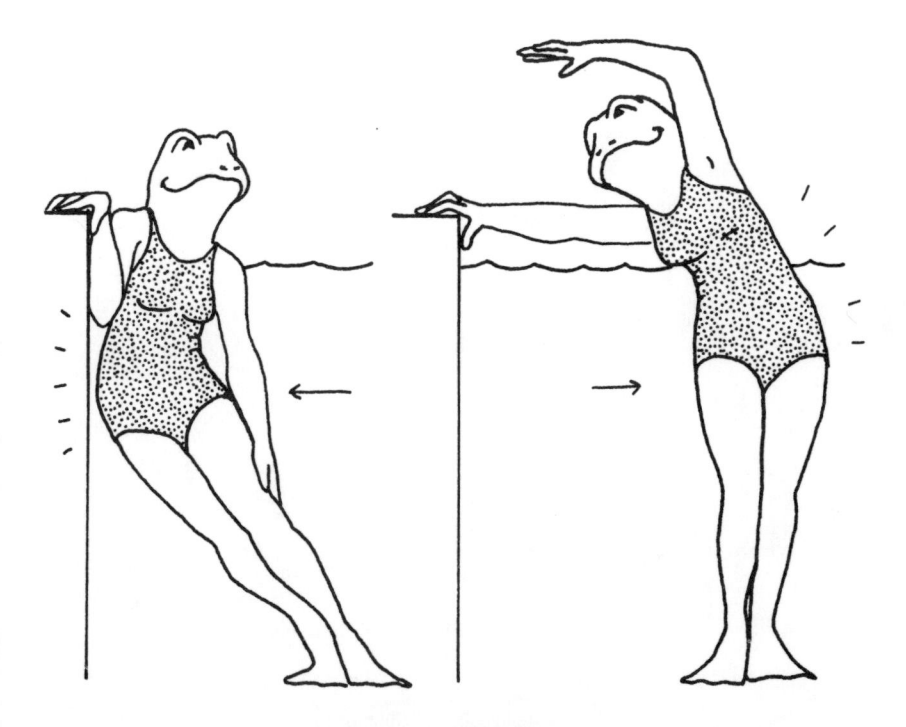

Tummy tucked
Bottom in
Stretch hips into the wall and away from the wall

KNEE TUCKS

Remember to keep your back against the wall

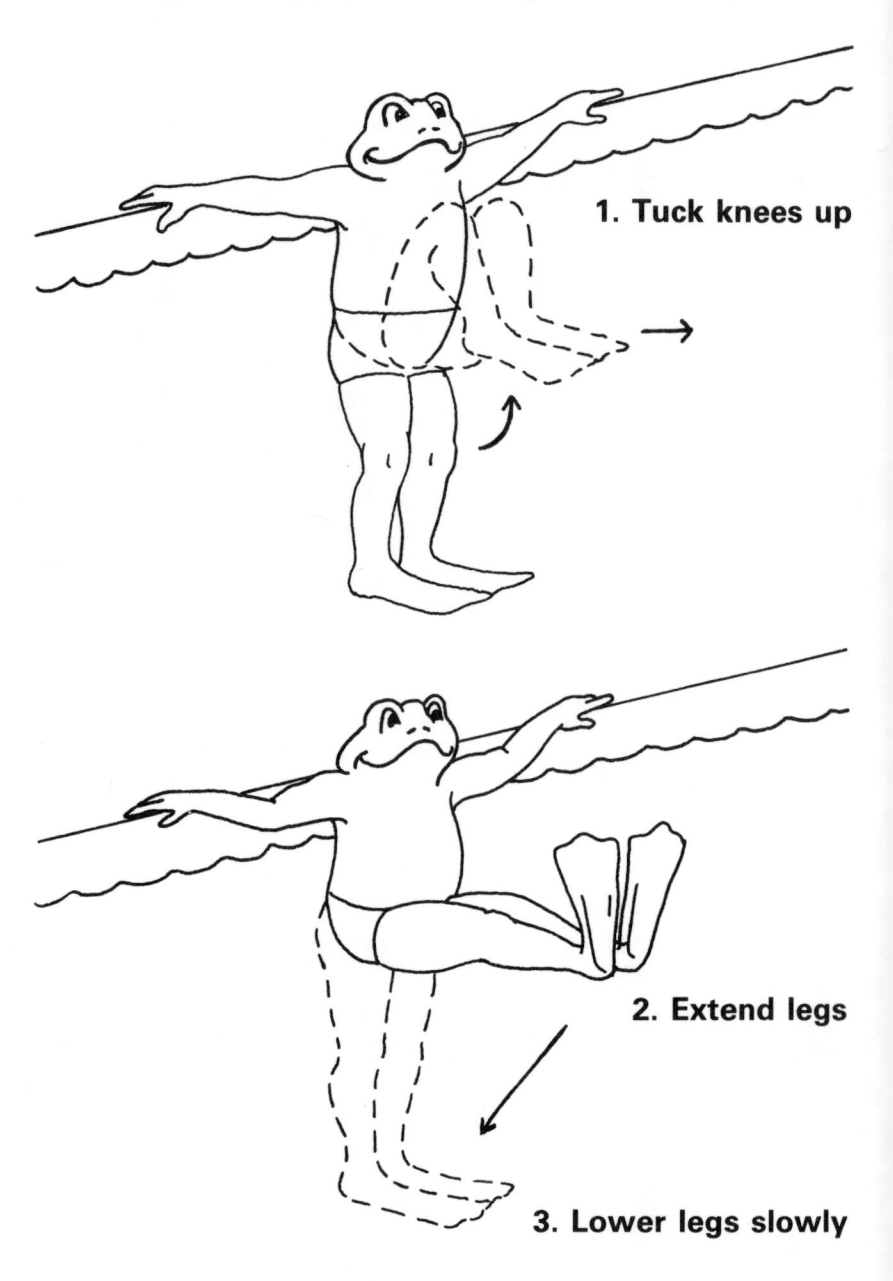

1. Tuck knees up

2. Extend legs

3. Lower legs slowly

36 WAIST AND ABDOMEN

LEG CIRCLES

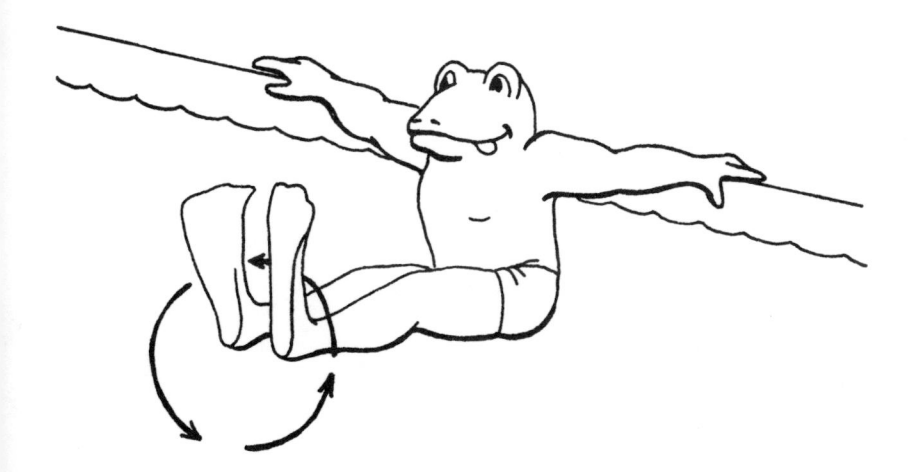

KNEE CIRCLES

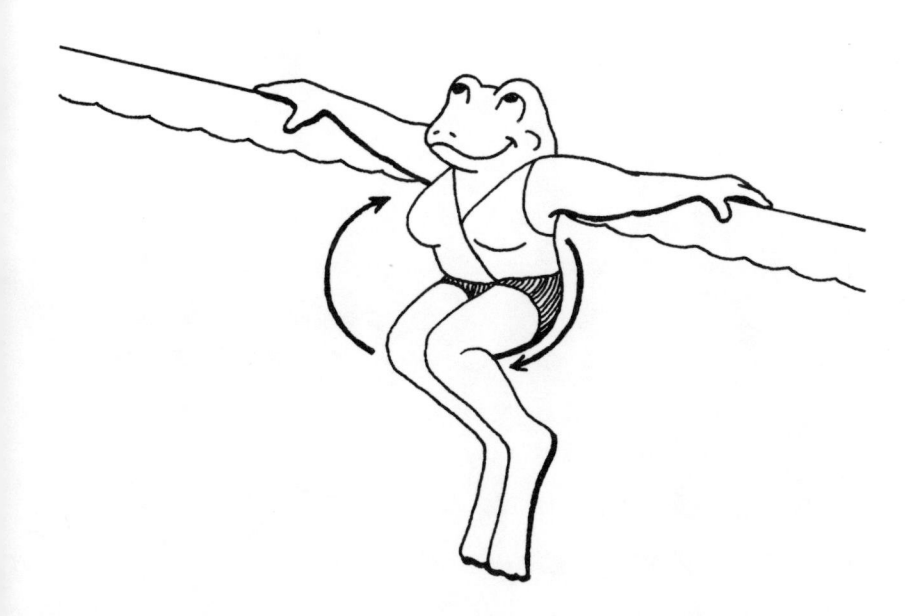

WAIST AND ABDOMEN

WINDSHIELD WIPERS
Swing legs right and left

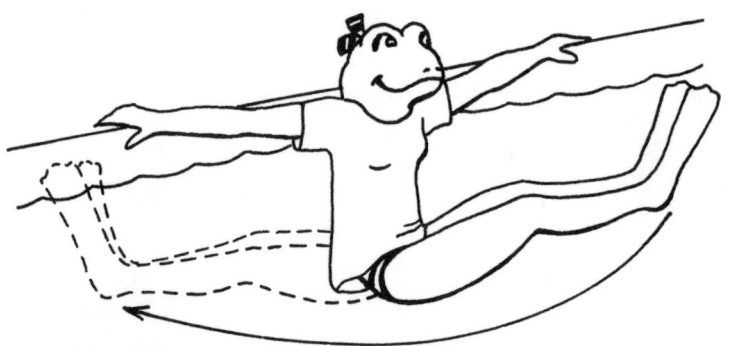

Legs together

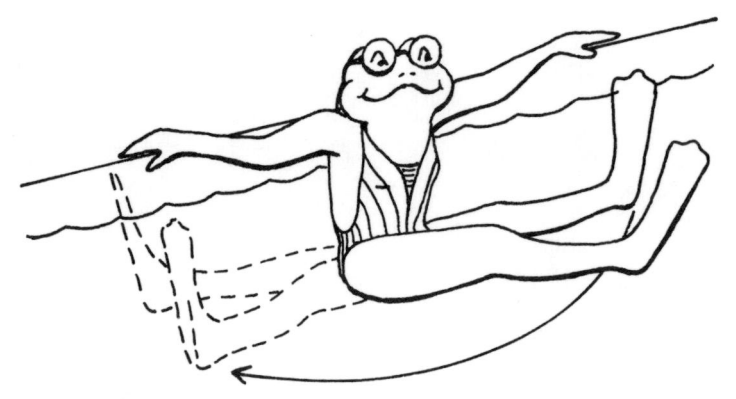

Legs 6" apart

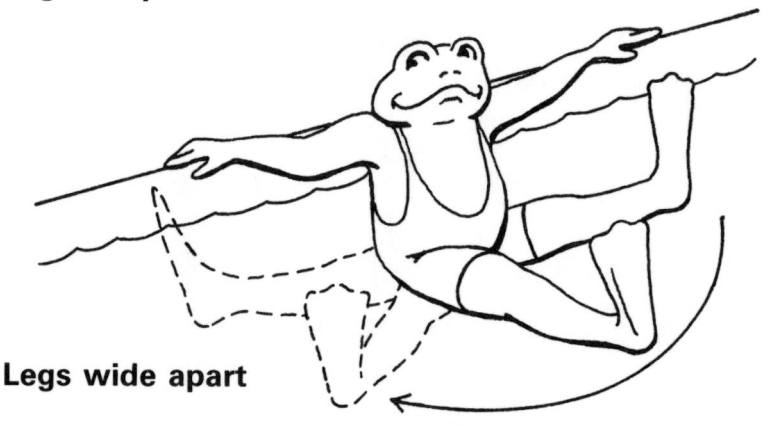

Legs wide apart

38 WAIST AND ABDOMEN

NOTES

**Do each position
5 times
then repeat the whole series
3 times**

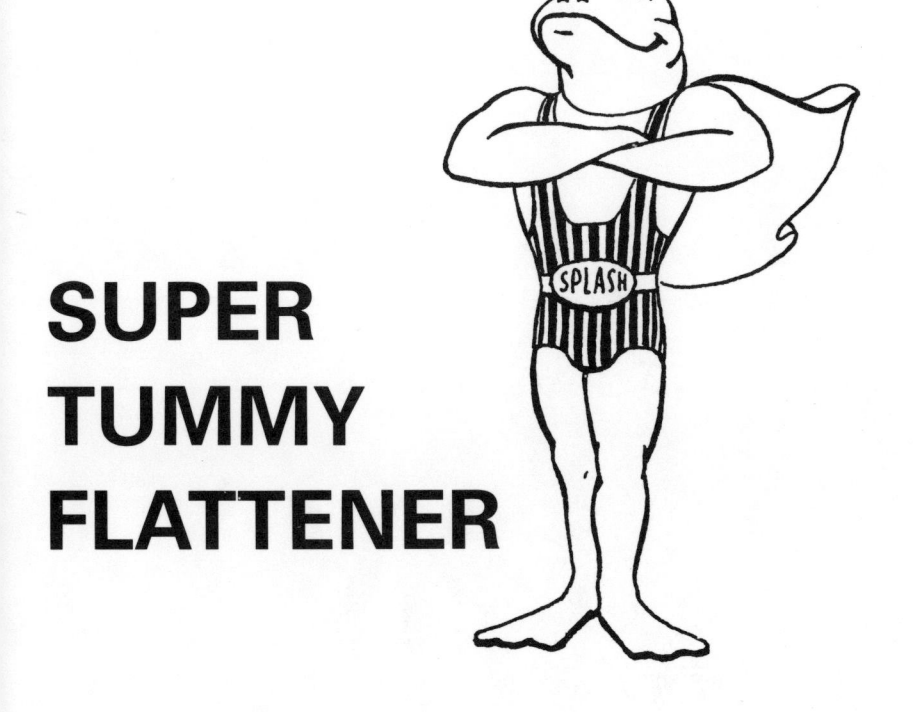

SUPER
TUMMY
FLATTENER

UP, UP - DOWN, DOWN HEELS ALWAYS ON THE FLOOR OR WALL

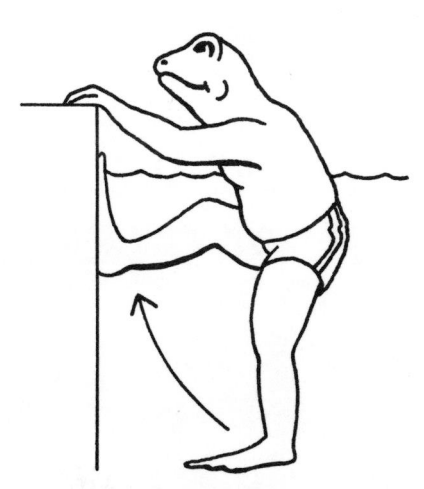

1. Right foot on the wall

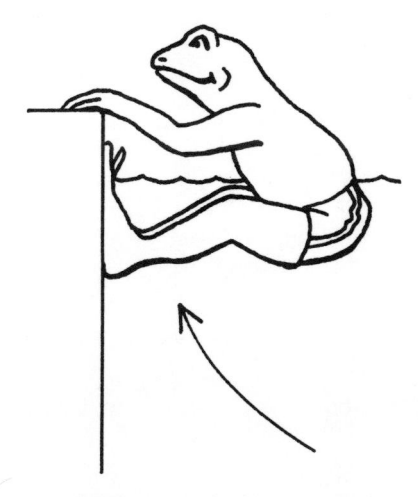

2. left foot on the wall

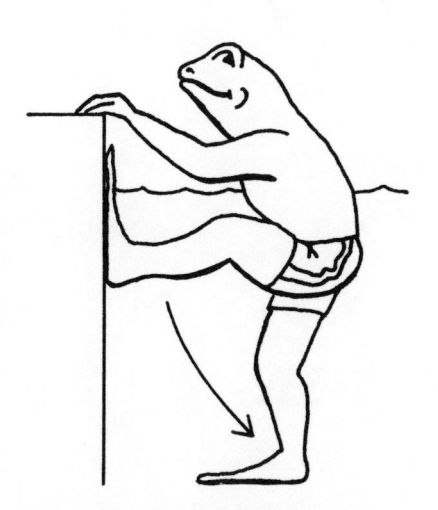

3. right foot to the floor

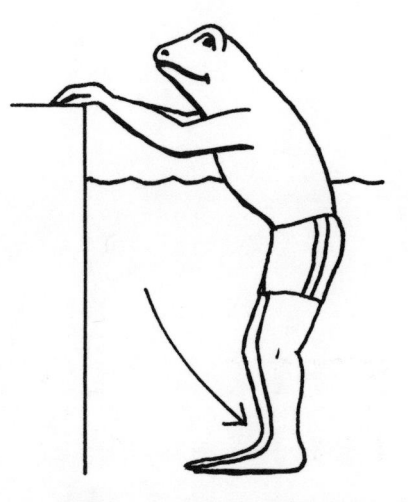

4. left foot to the floor

SUPER TUMMY FLATTENER

FEET RIGHT AND LEFT

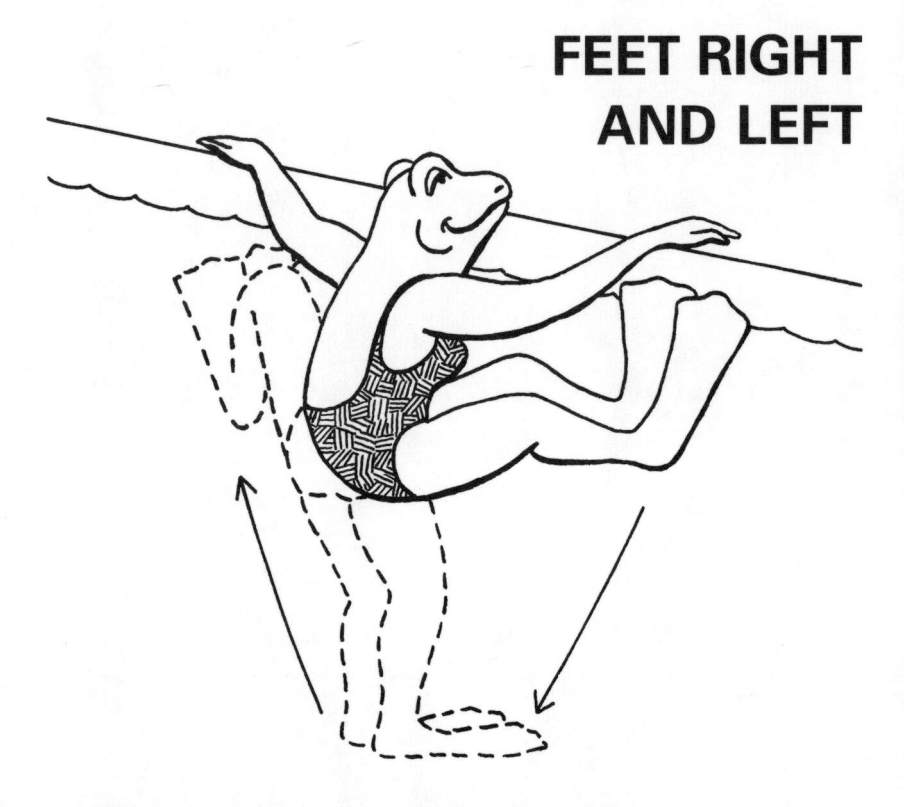

FEET ON FLOOR THEN FEET ON WALL

44 SUPER TUMMY FLATTENER

BOTH FEET TOGETHER

ON WALL THEN ON FLOOR

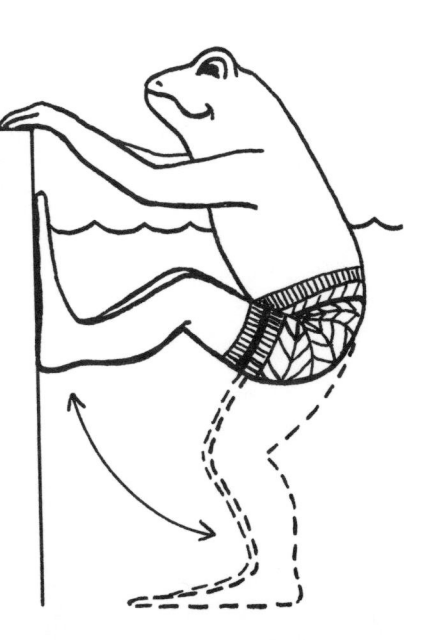

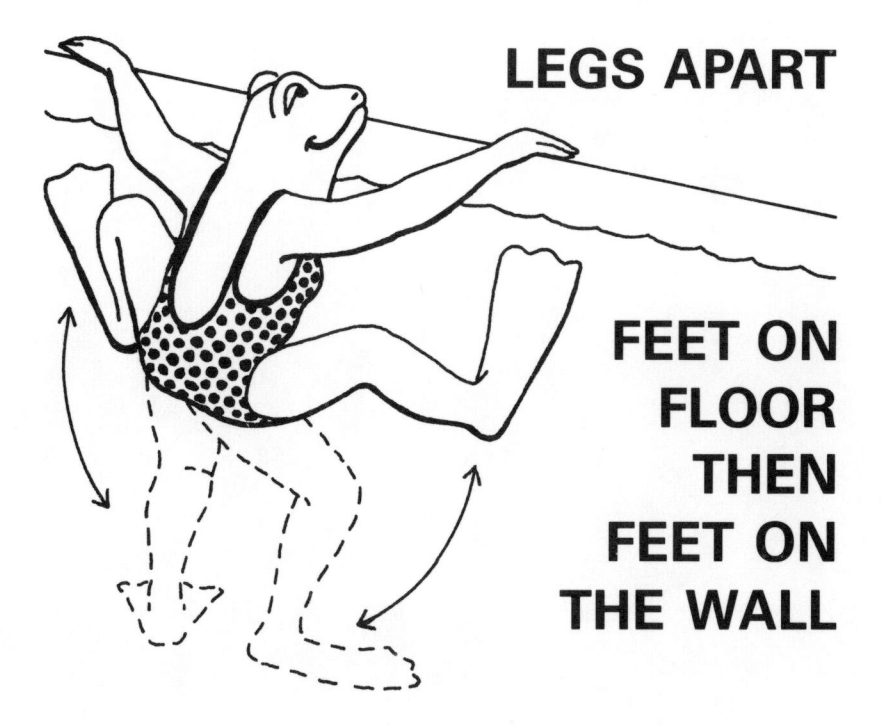

LEGS APART

FEET ON FLOOR THEN FEET ON THE WALL

SUPER TUMMY FLATTENER 45

THIGHS AND HIPS

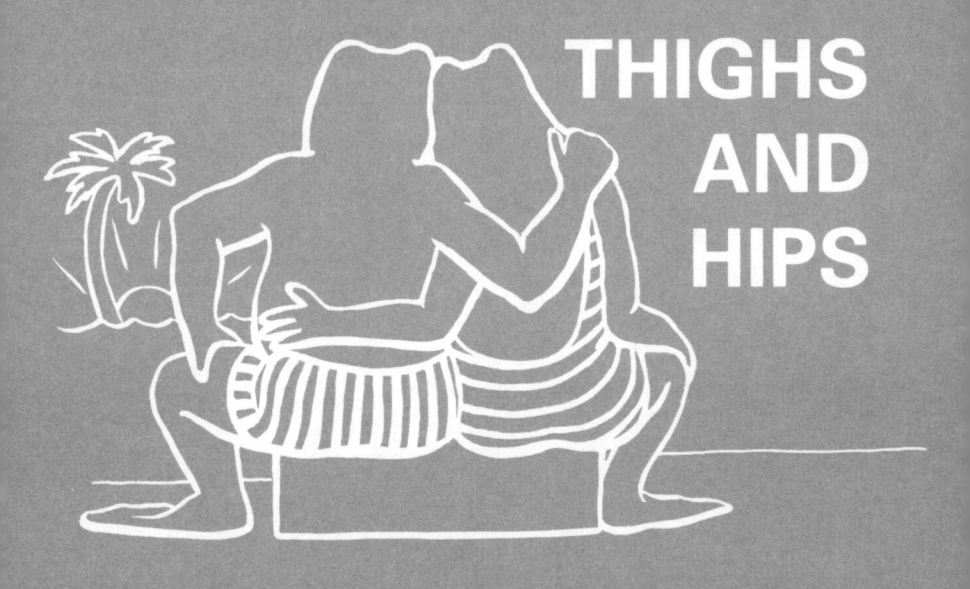

PIGEON TOES

Back snug to wall
Turn toes in
Heels lead moving whole leg out and in

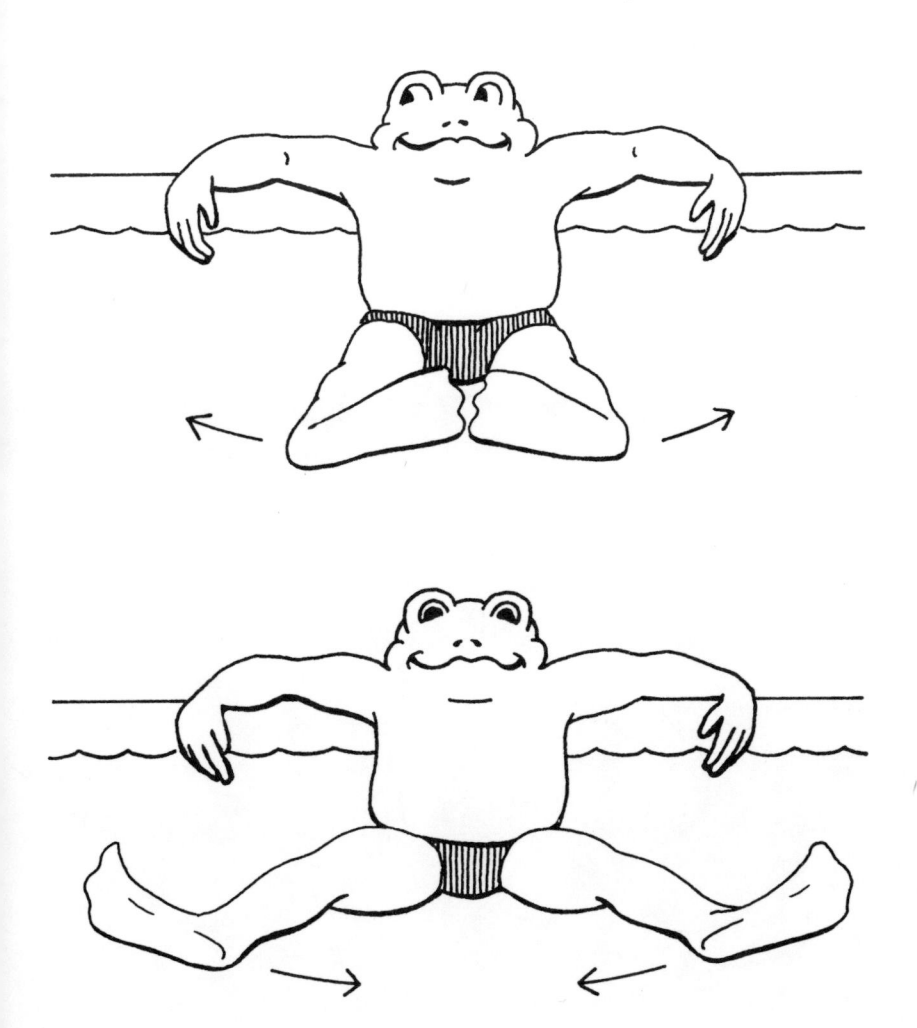

THIGHS AND HIPS

PULSES

Do little pulses with legs in apart position

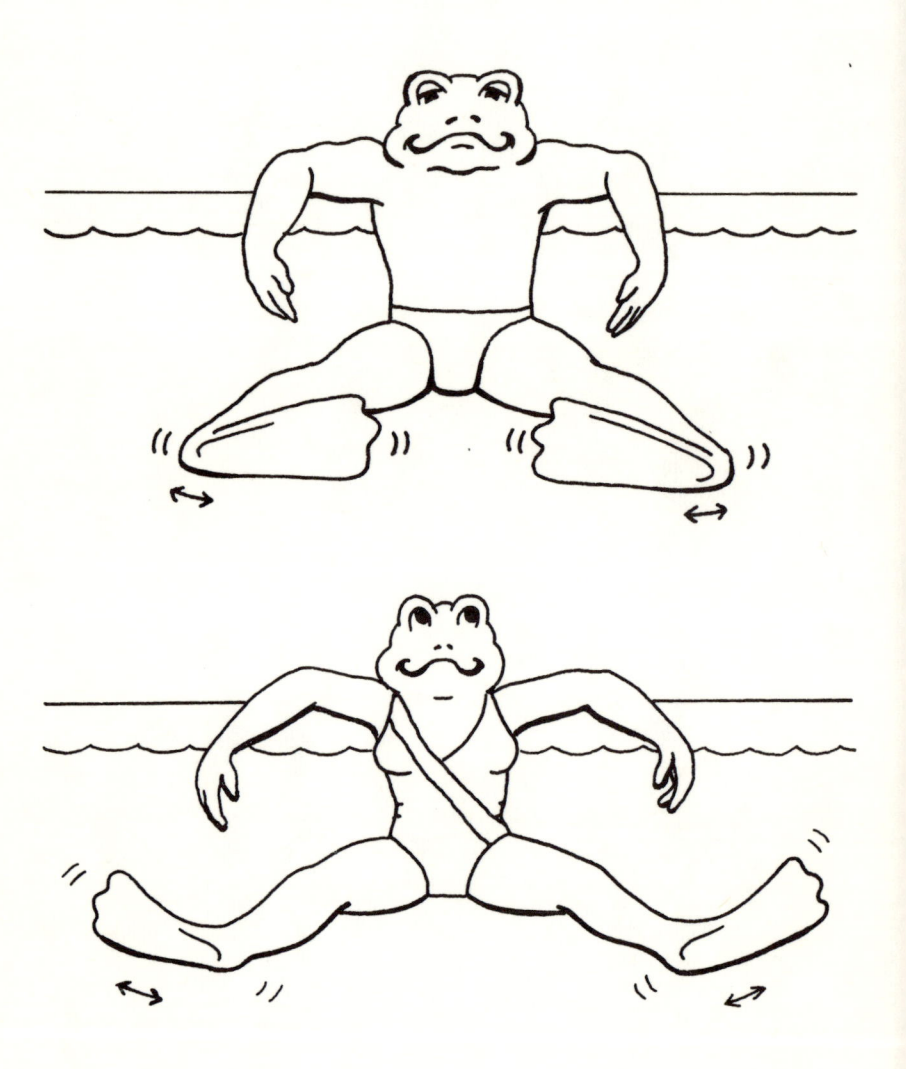

50 THIGHS AND HIPS

BIG THEN LITTLE CRISS-CROSSES

Do 5 wide leg criss-crosses then 5 small criss-crosses (crossing at the ankles)

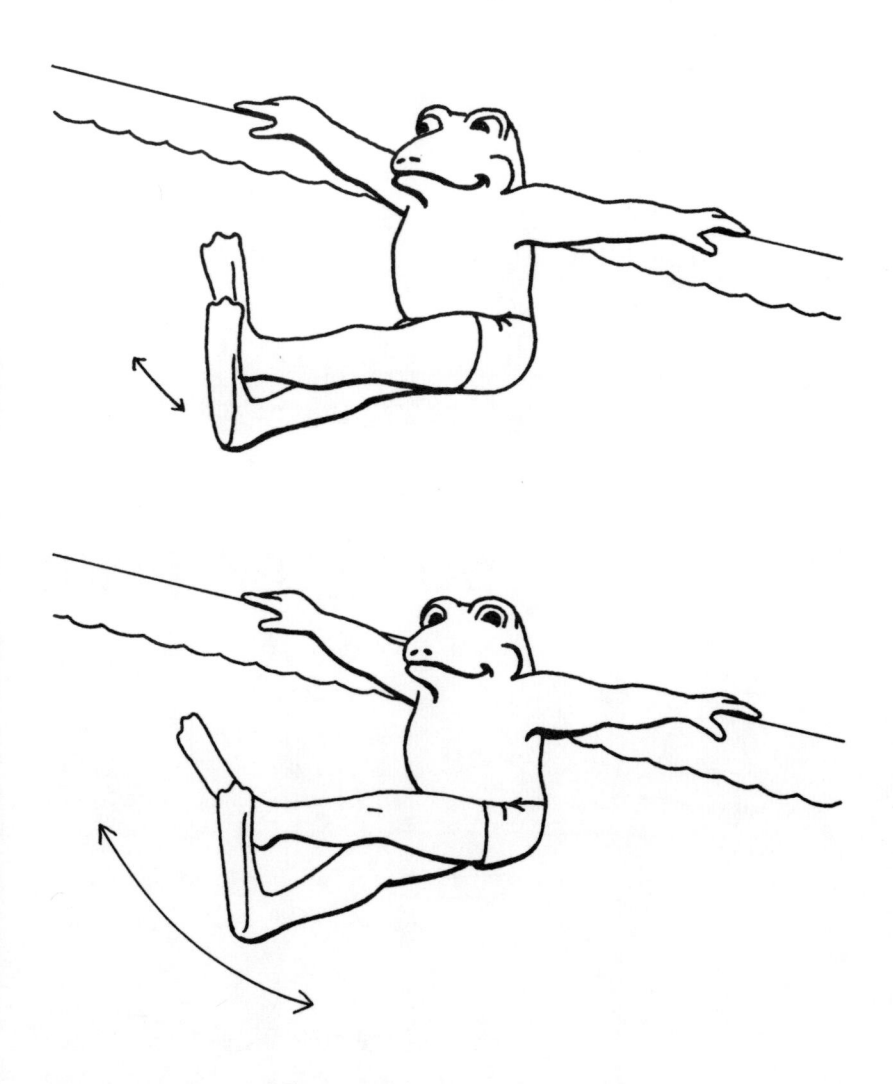

FLOOR TOUCHES

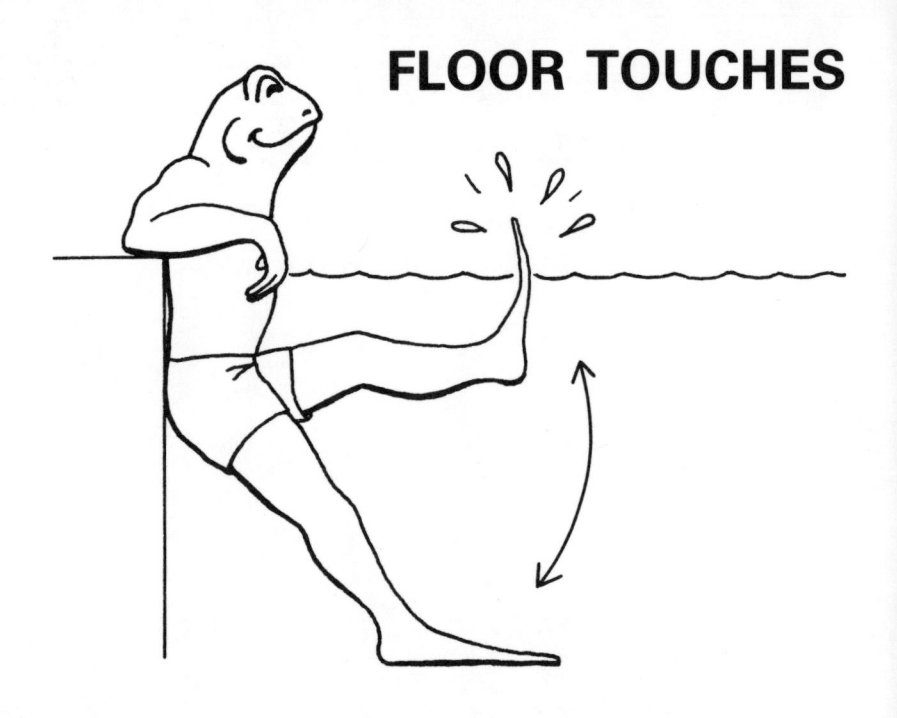

NOWHERE KICKS

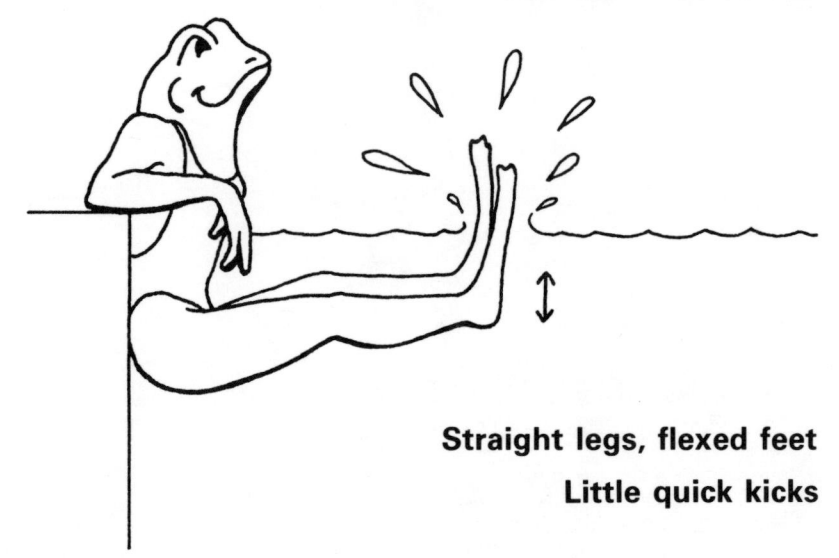

Straight legs, flexed feet
Little quick kicks

52 THIGHS AND HIPS

FLOOR TOUCHES II

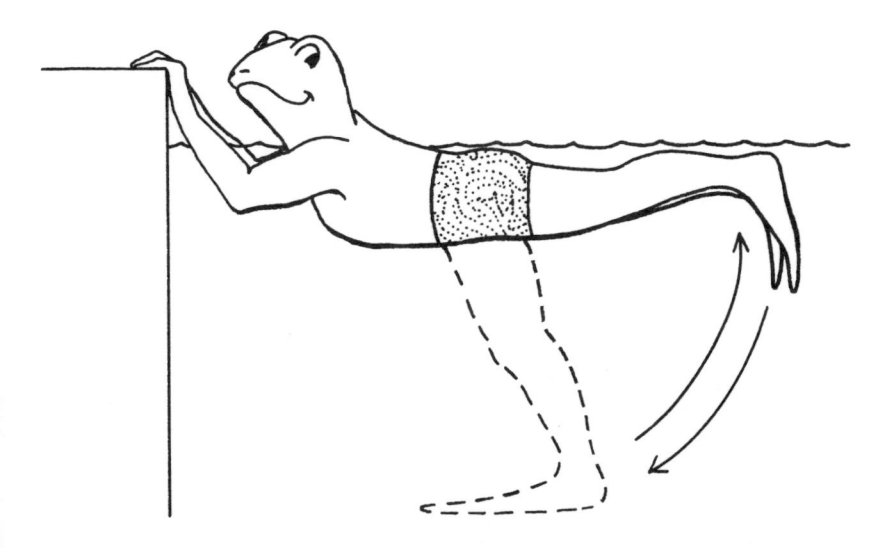

Alternate foot touching floor

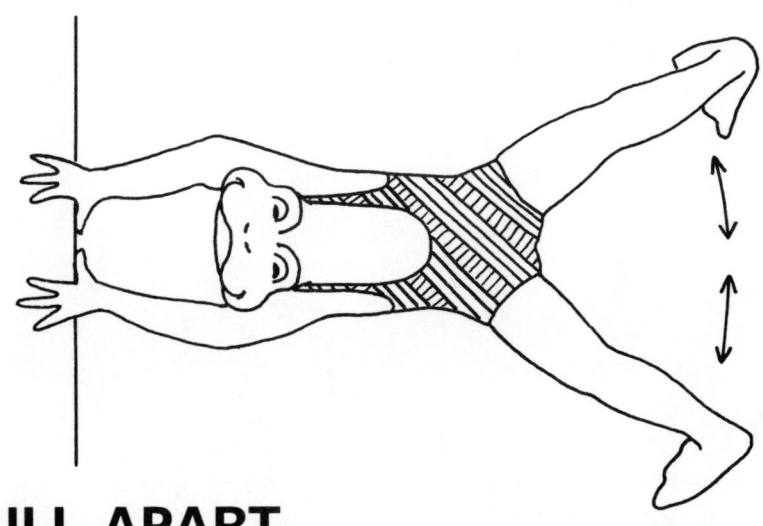

PULL APART

Straight legs   Take legs wide apart and back together

THIGHS AND HIPS 53

FORWARD LEG SWING

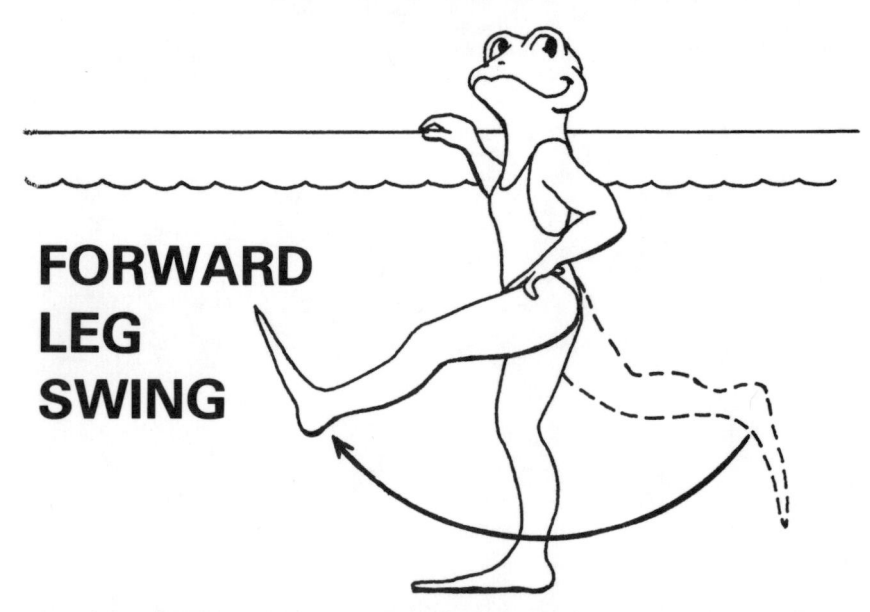

**Stand tall (bottom tucked, tummy in) side to wall
Swing outside leg forward and back**

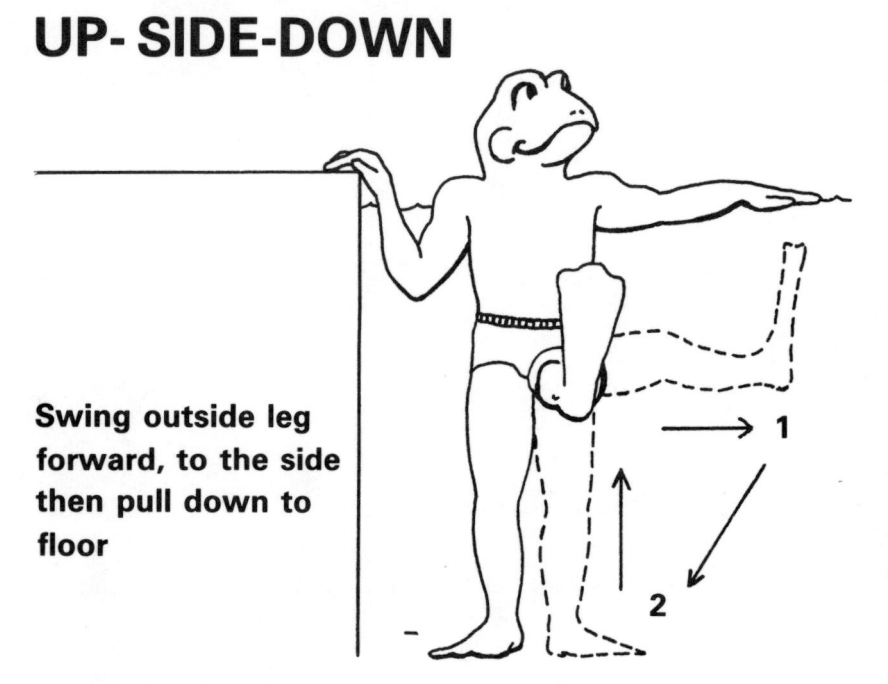

UP-SIDE-DOWN

Swing outside leg forward, to the side then pull down to floor

54 THIGHS AND HIPS

SIDE SWEEP

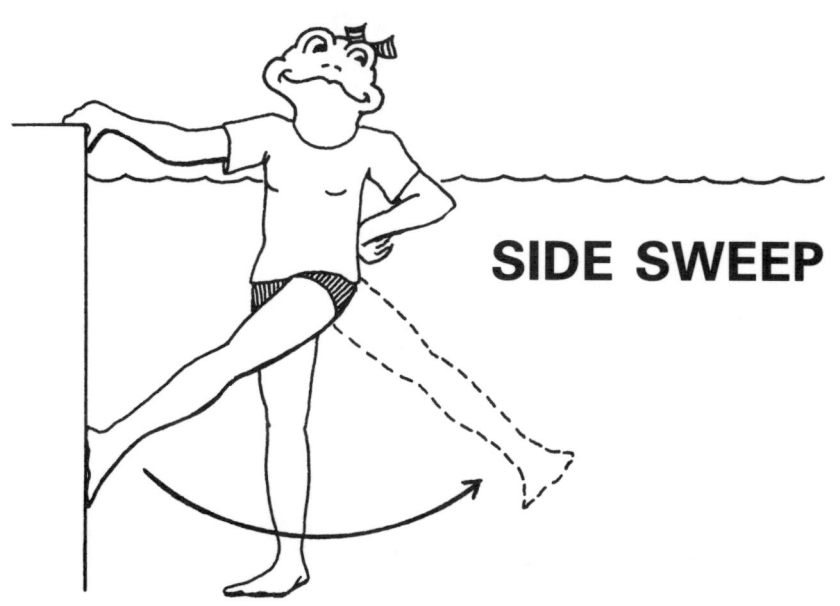

Cross foot in front of body to wall then swing out

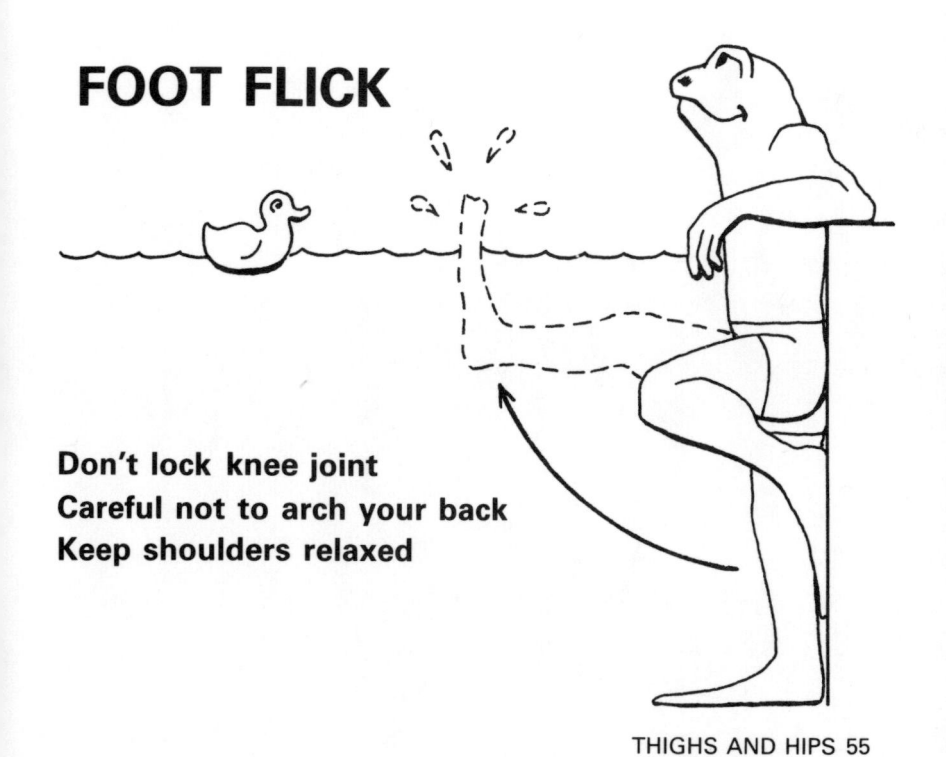

FOOT FLICK

Don't lock knee joint
Careful not to arch your back
Keep shoulders relaxed

"V" LEGS

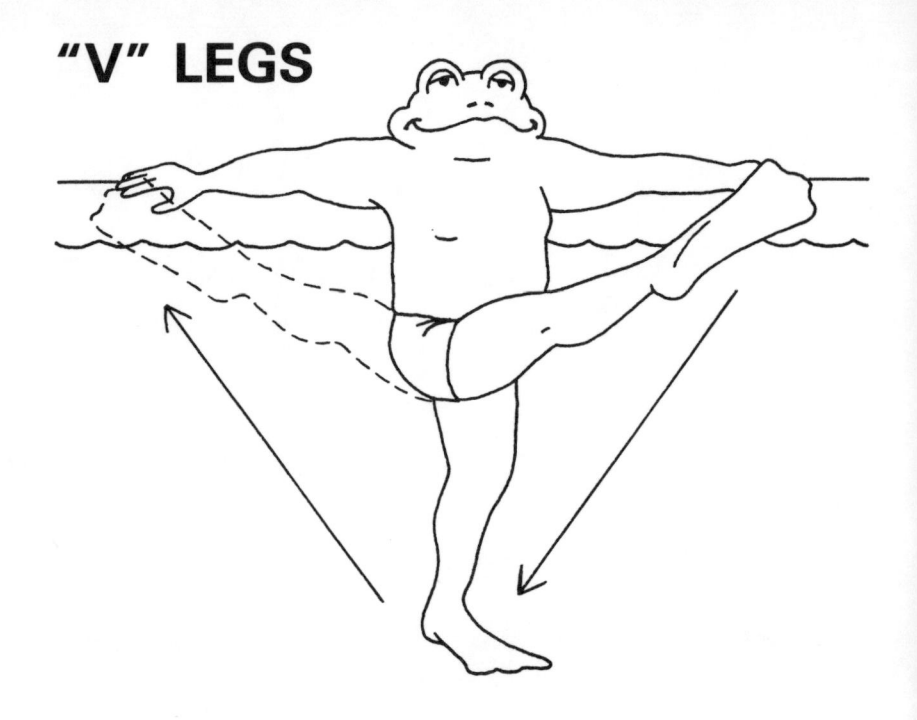

HINGE KICK

Careful not to arch back

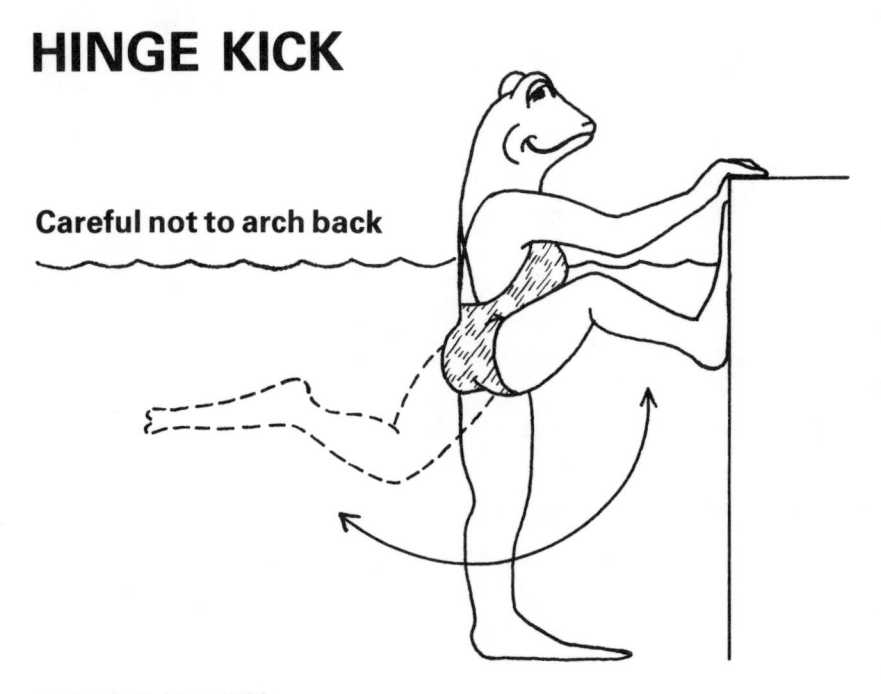

56 THIGHS AND HIPS

BICYCLES

One hip to the surface for awhile then the other

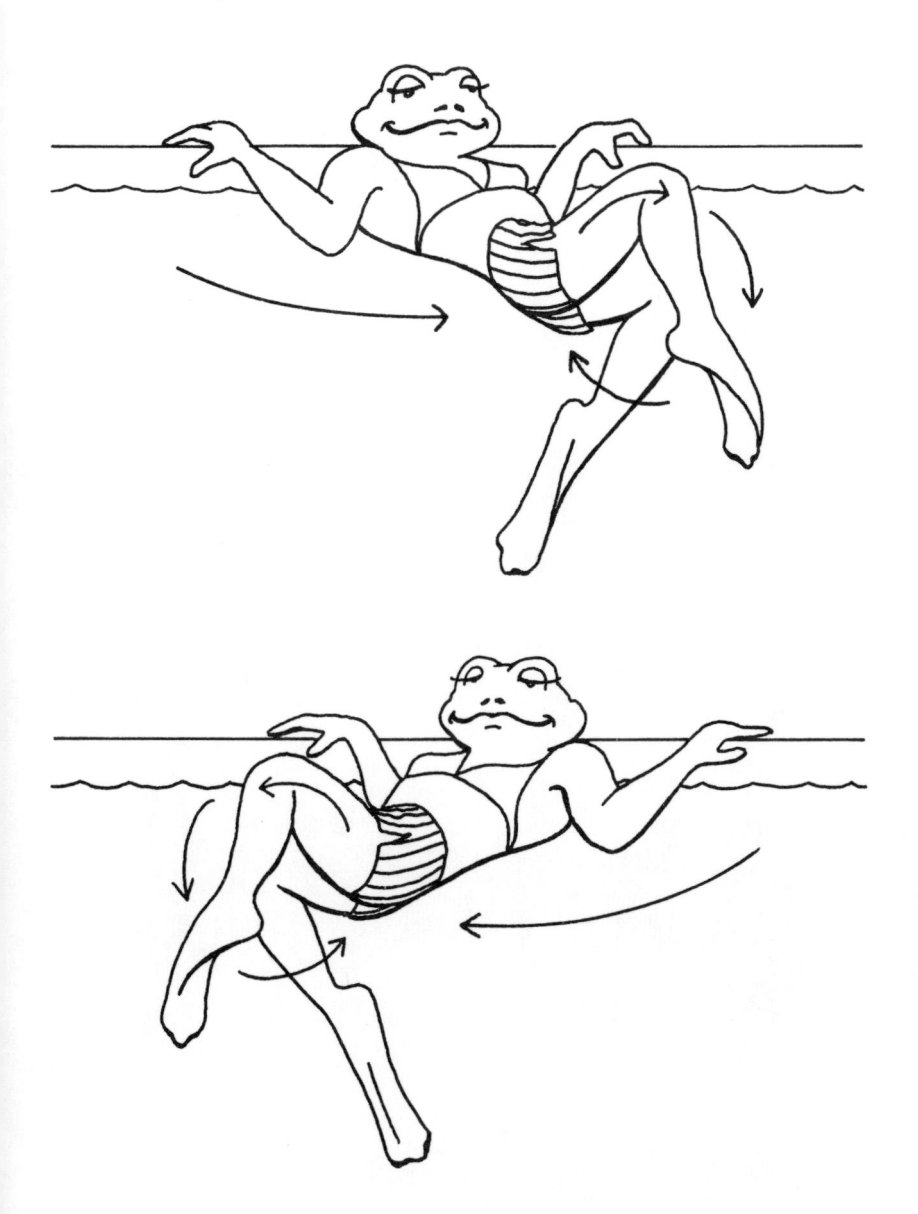

THIGHS AND HIPS

DOGGIE AND VARIATIONS

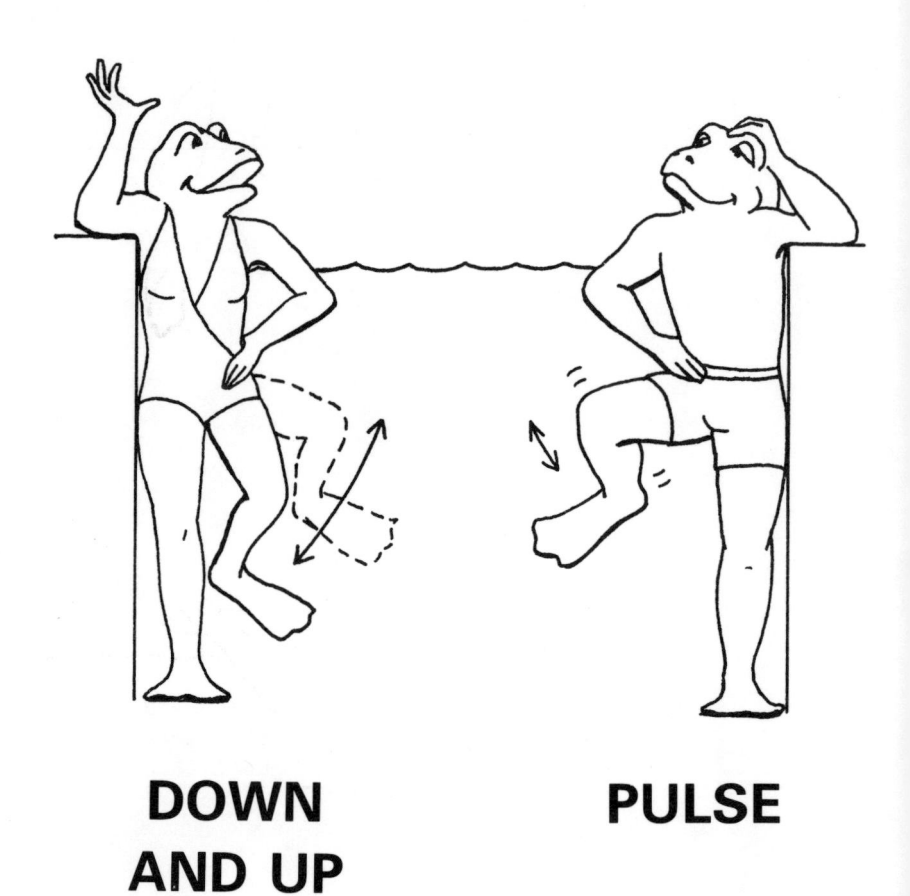

DOWN AND UP **PULSE**

58 THIGHS AND HIPS

All "Doggie" (hip and thigh) exercises done at the wall may also be done by holding onto the jugs, just remember to keep good posture and to bend your standing knee slightly.

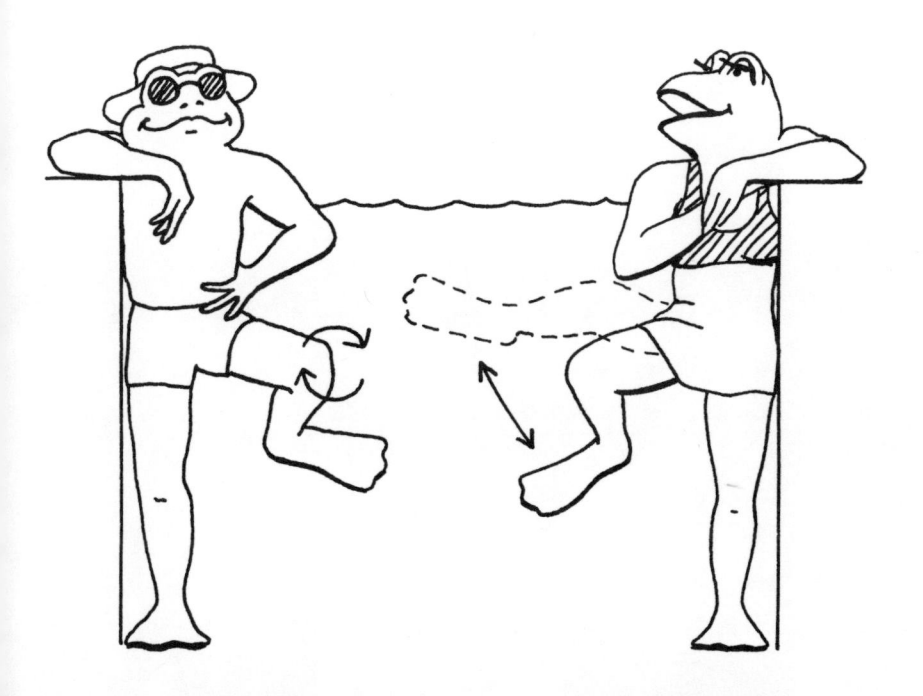

HIP ISOLATION

KARATE KICK

THIGHS AND HIPS

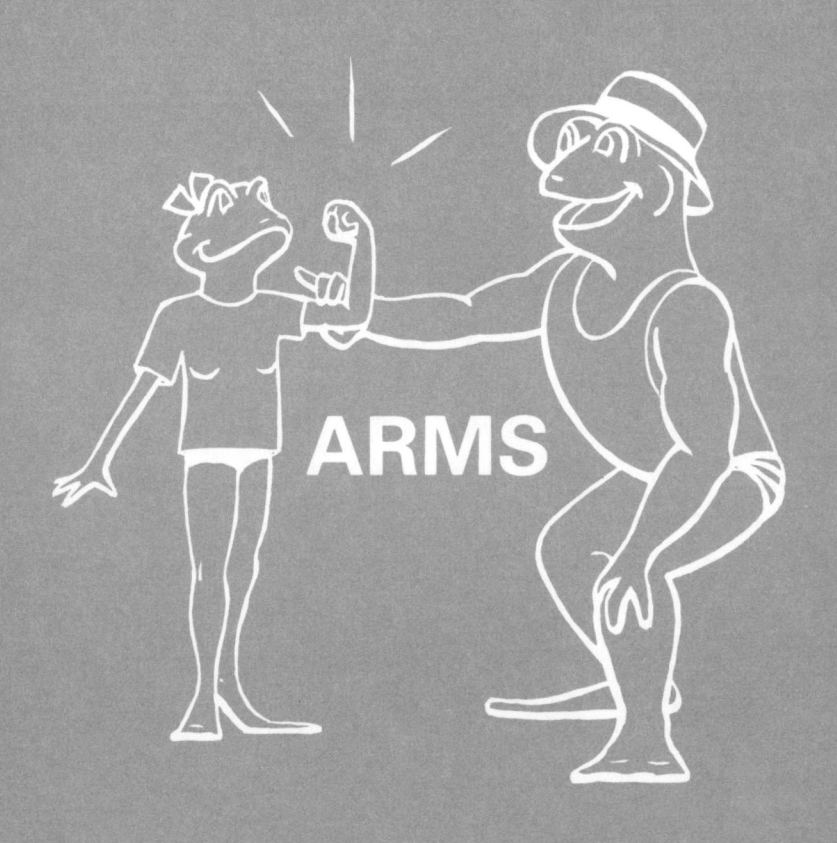

ARMS

BIG CIRCLES

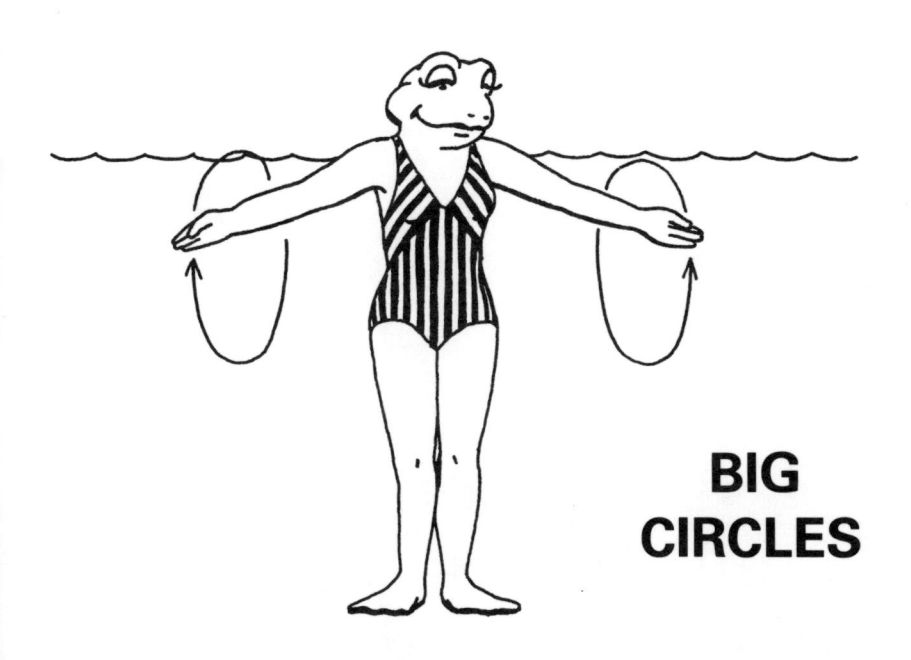

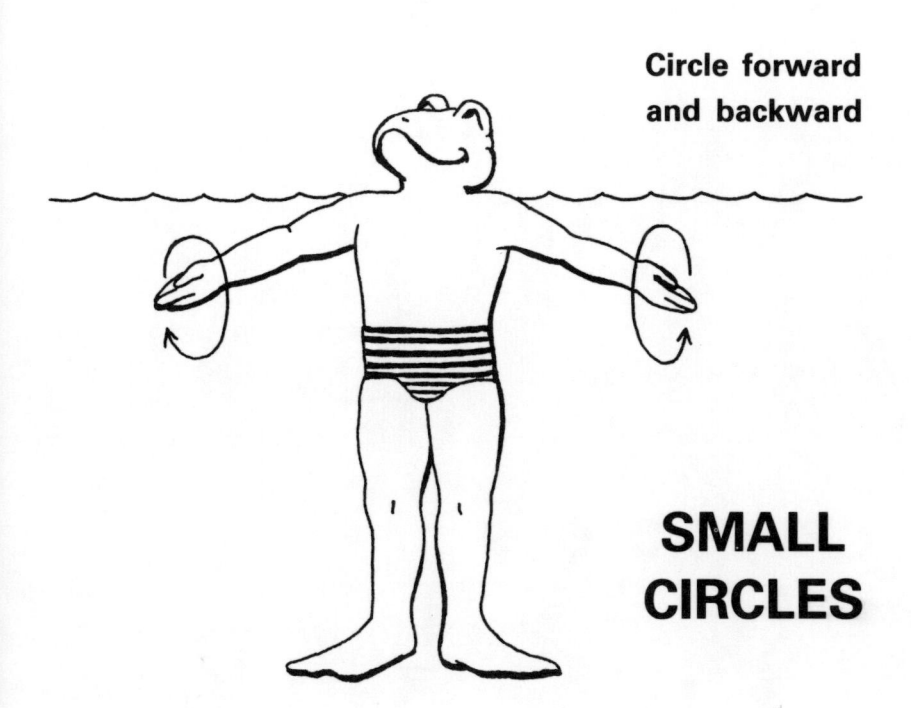

Circle forward and backward

SMALL CIRCLES

ARMS 63

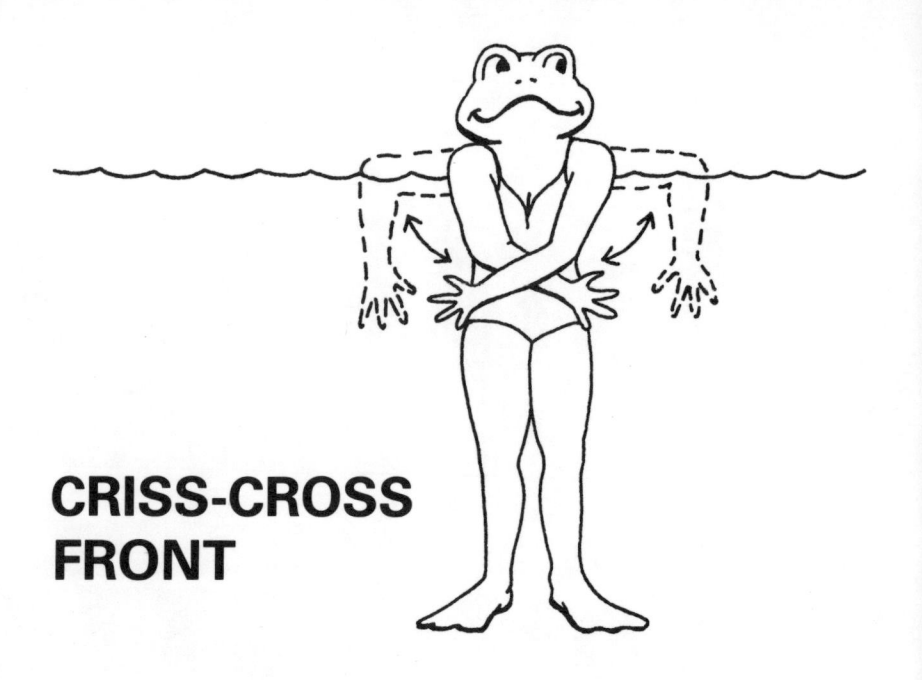

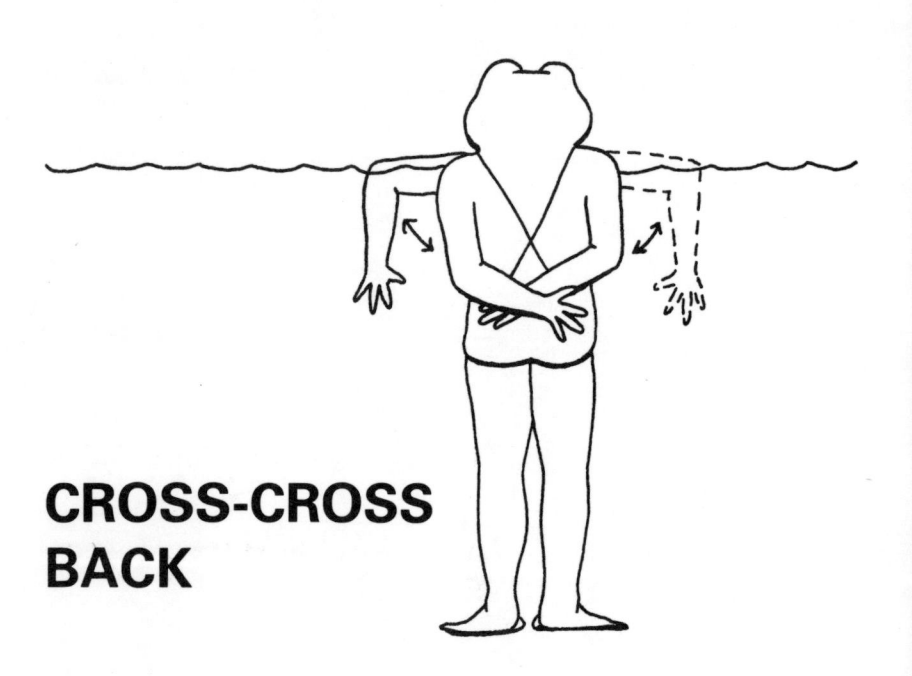

CRISS-CROSS FRONT

CROSS-CROSS BACK

FRONT CLAPS

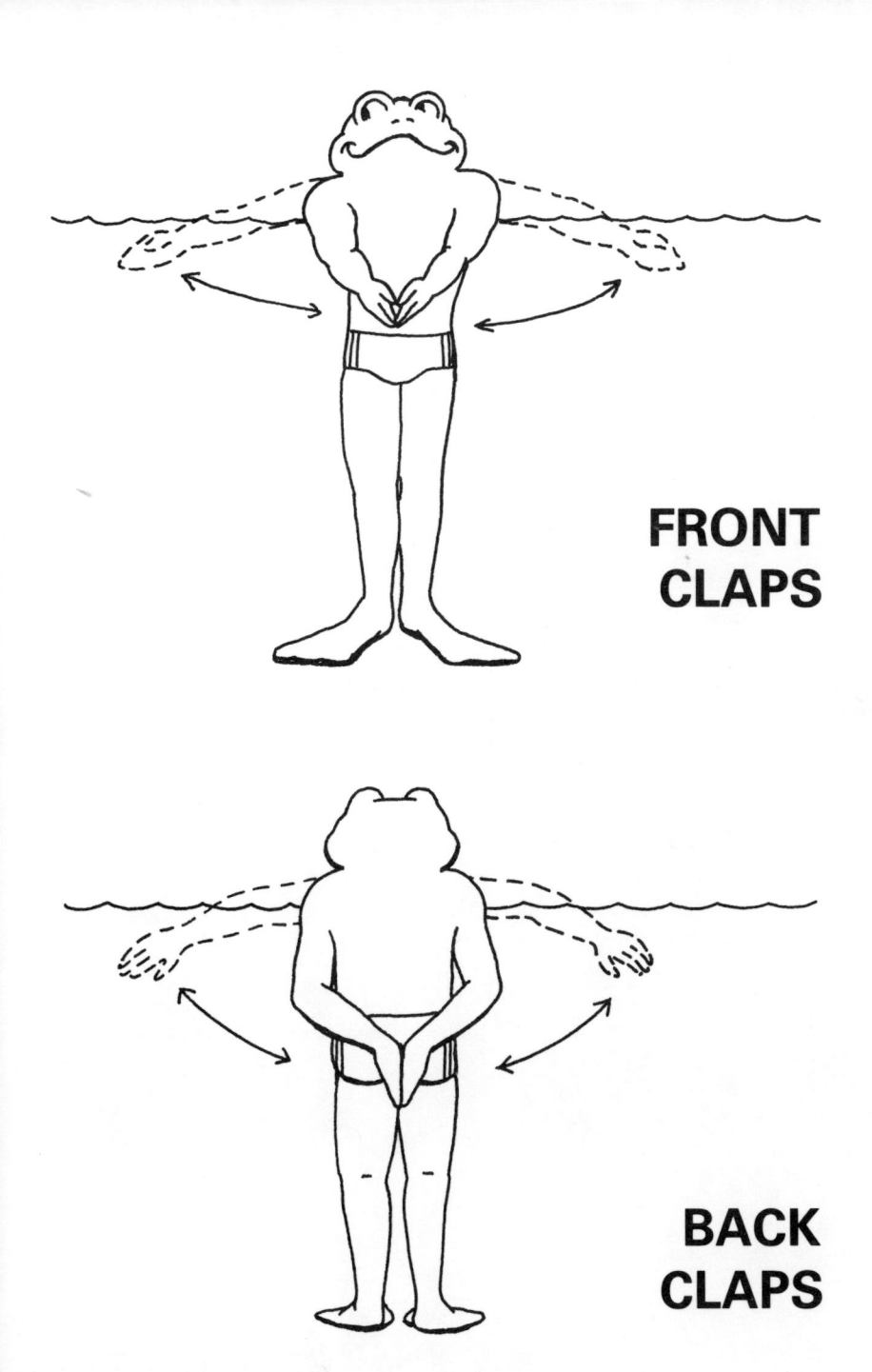

BACK CLAPS

ARMS 65

Palms down

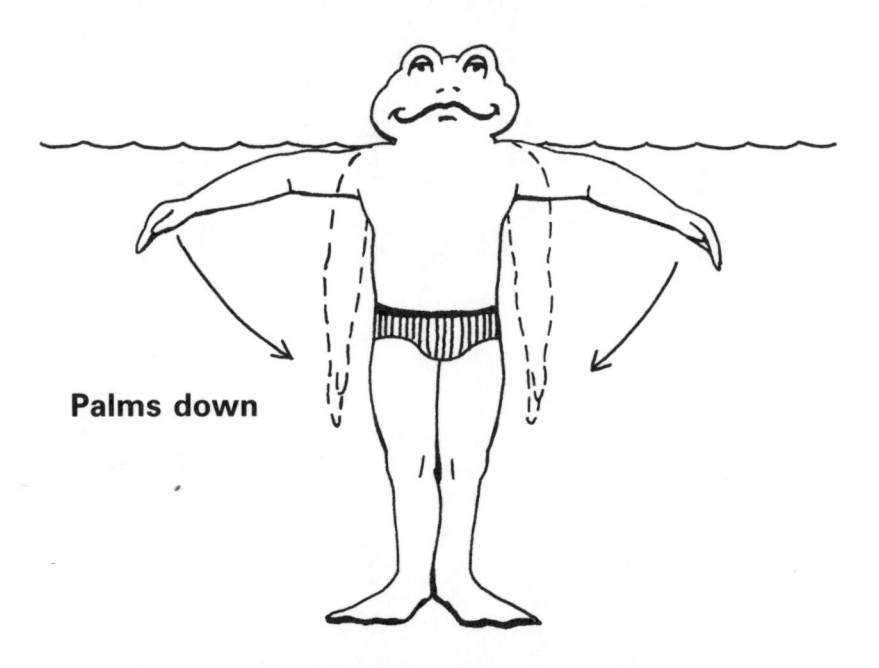

DOWN AND UP

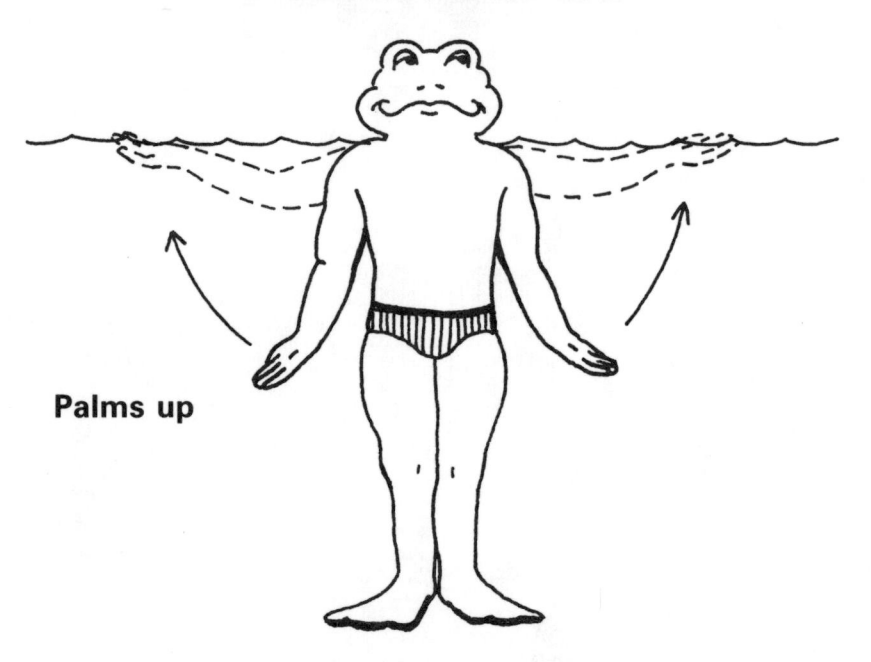

Palms up

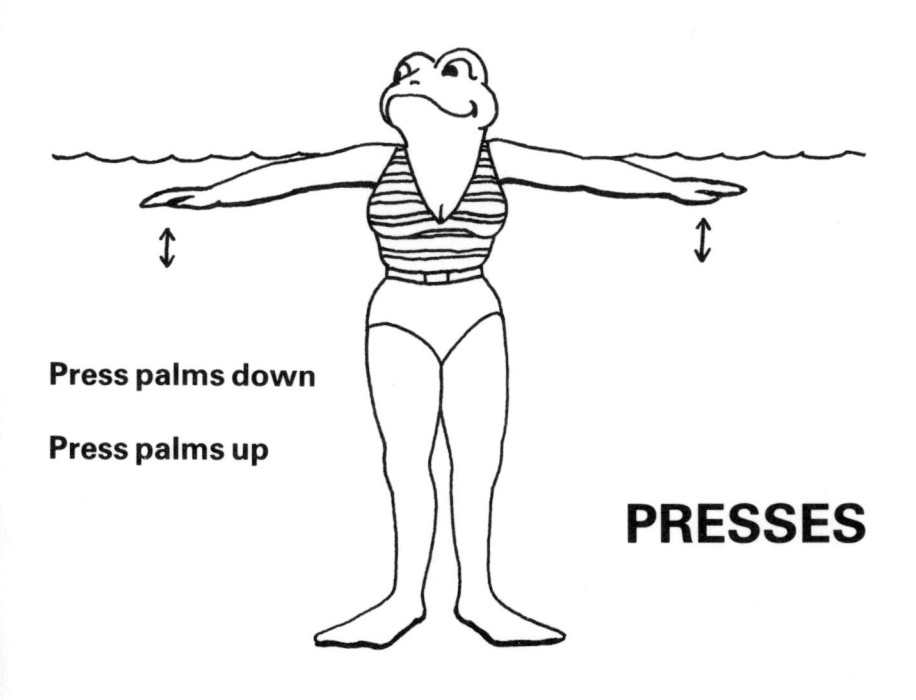

Press palms down

Press palms up

PRESSES

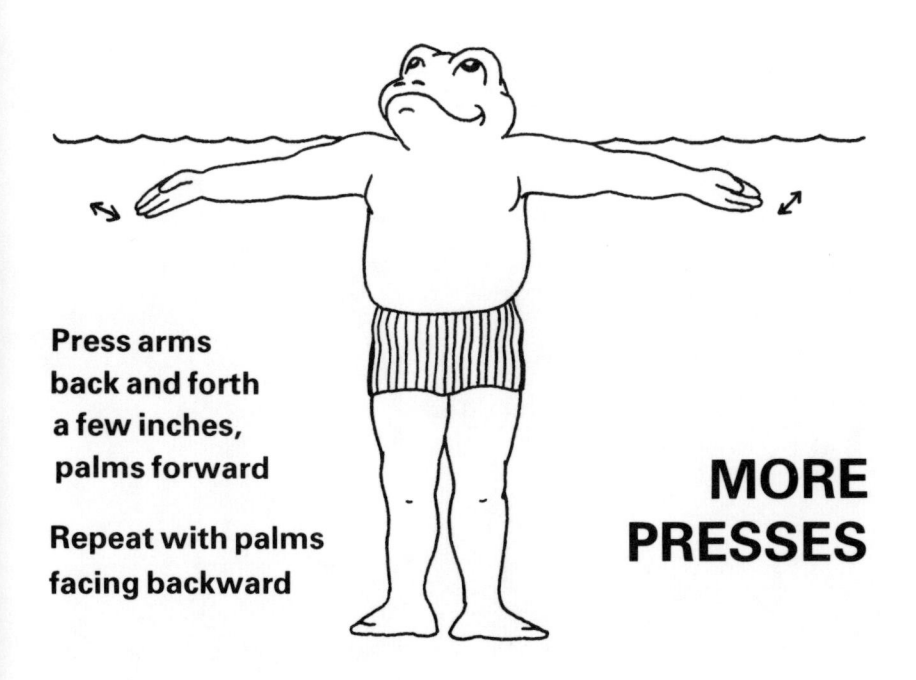

Press arms back and forth a few inches, palms forward

Repeat with palms facing backward

MORE PRESSES

67 ARMS

DOOR KNOB TURNS

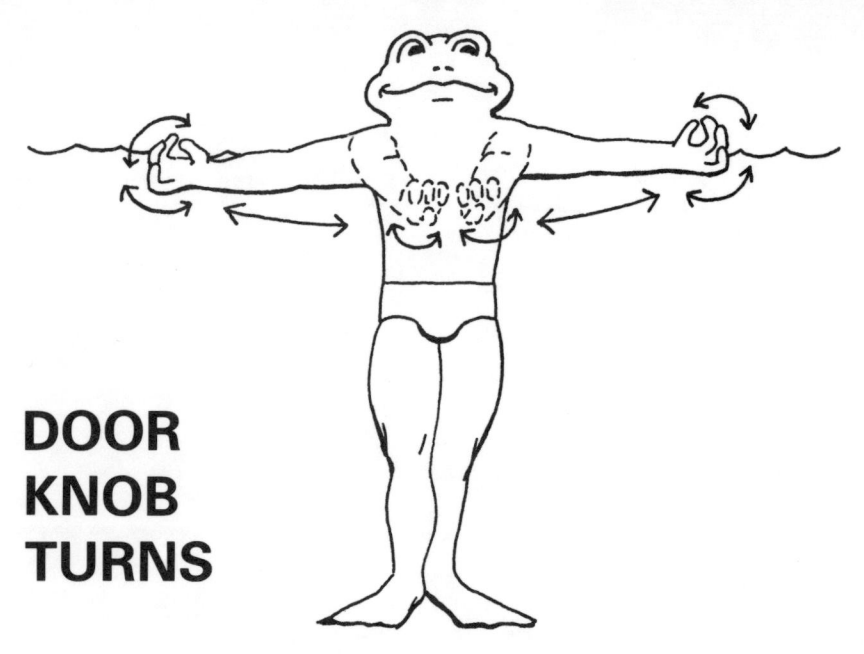

Roll hands forward and backwards

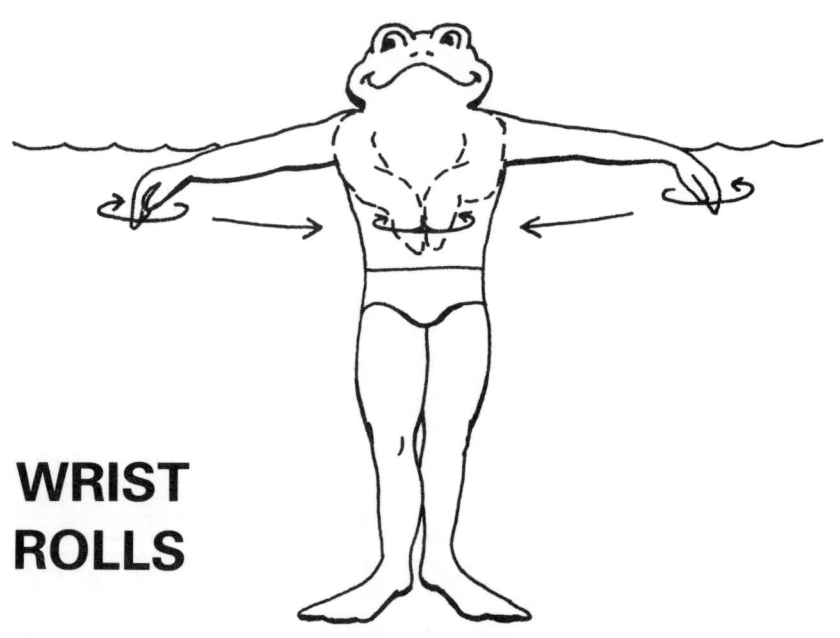

WRIST ROLLS

Stir hands forward   Stir hands back to starting position

PRESS AND LIFT

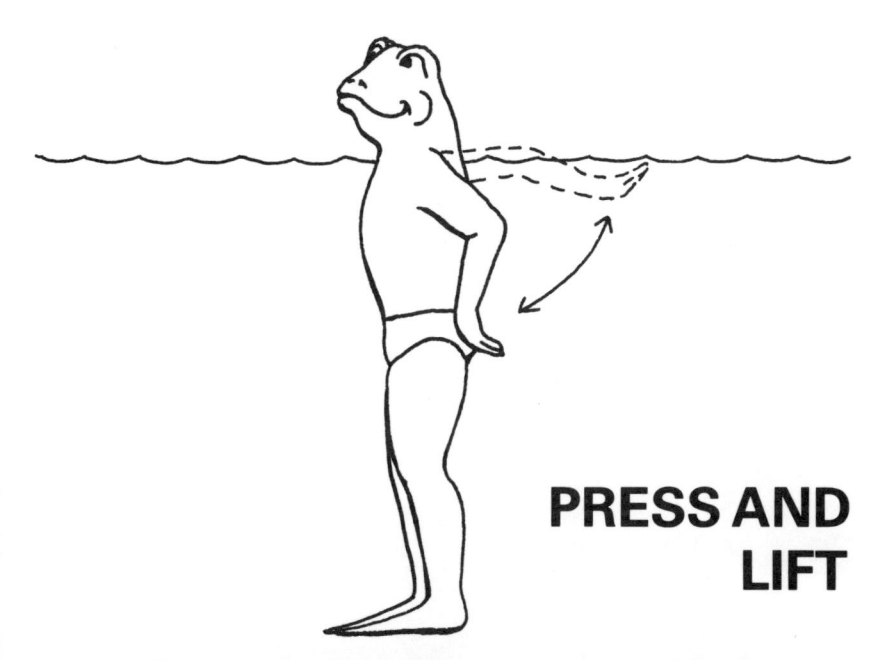

**Hands against bottom, palms turned out
Lift arms up and return to starting position**

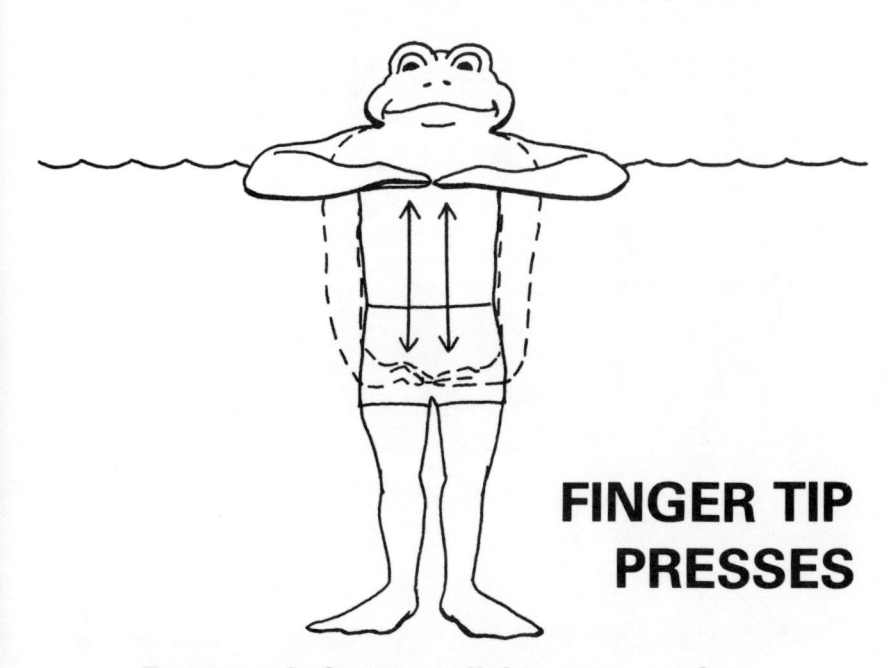

FINGER TIP PRESSES

Forearms in front parallel to water surface

ARMS 69

BACK HAND CLAPS

Forearms in front parallel to water surface

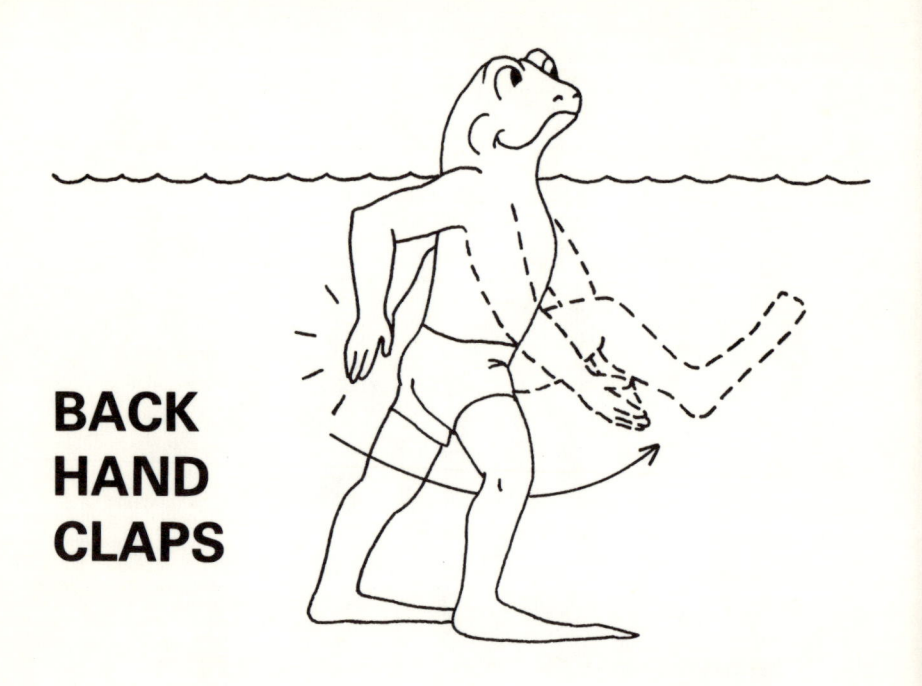

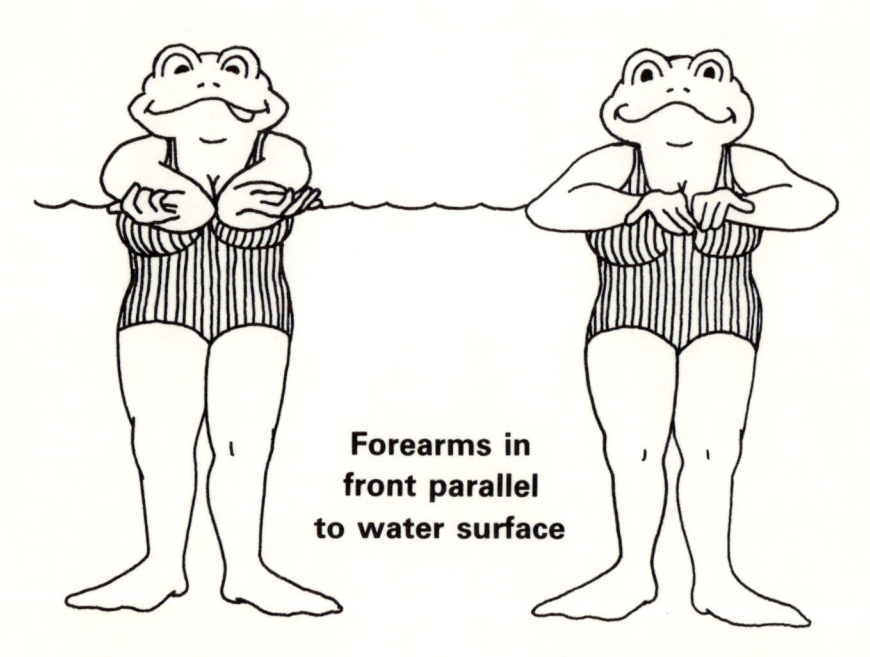

Take wrists apart (elbows together)

Take elbows apart (wrists together)

70 ARMS

PUSH-UPS

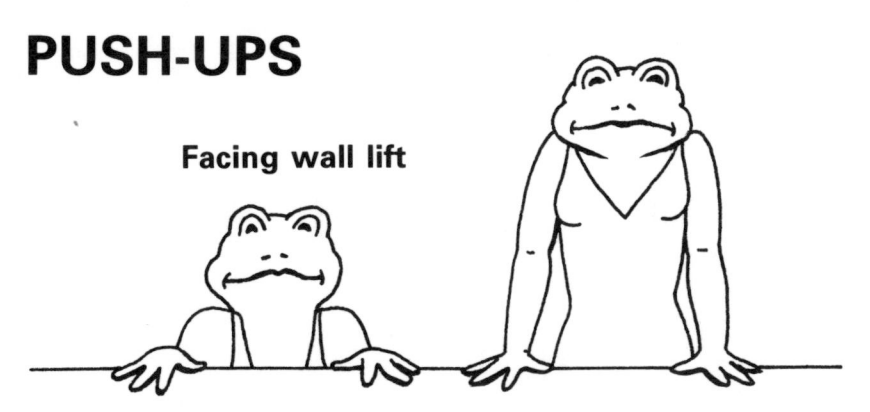

Facing wall lift

Lift to the count of 3   Hold 3 counts
Lower to the count of 5

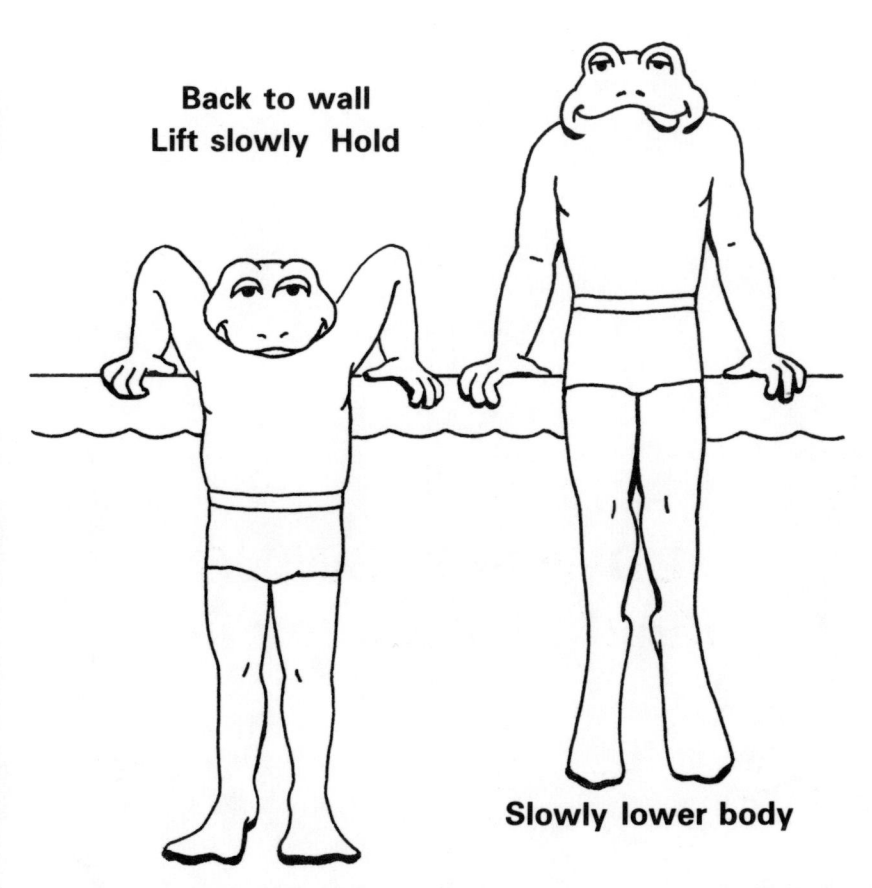

Back to wall
Lift slowly Hold

Slowly lower body

ARMS 71

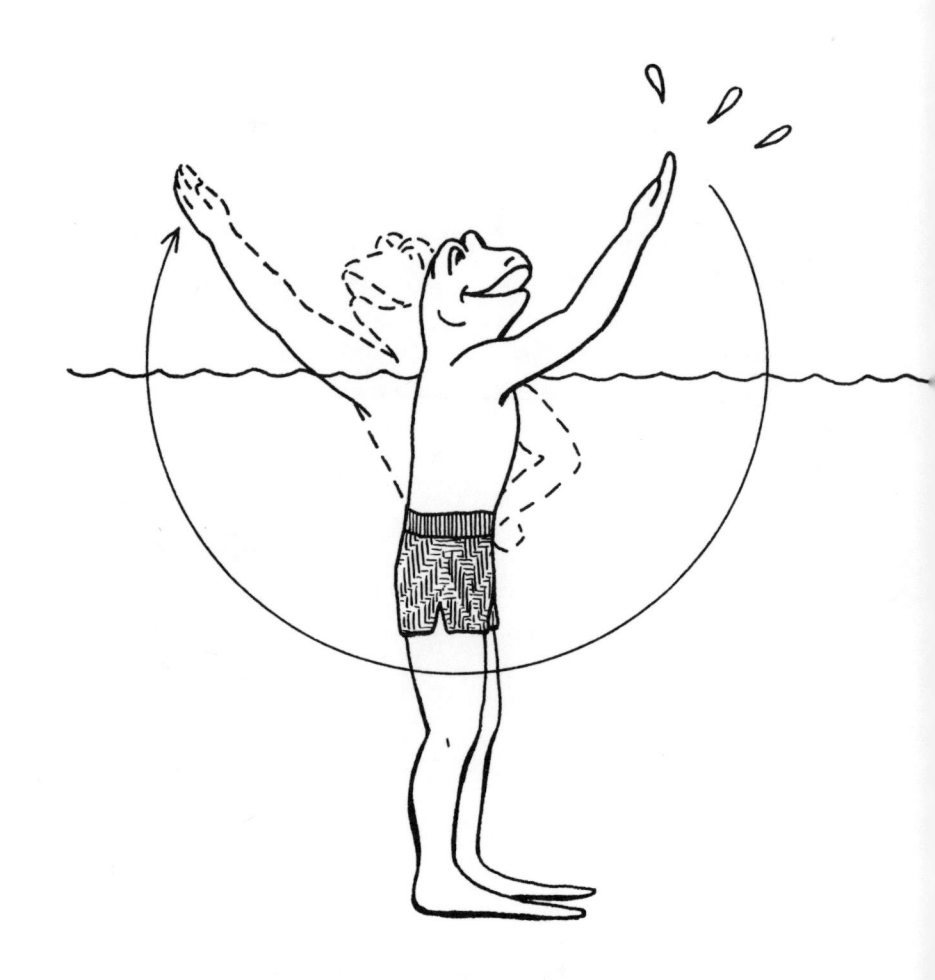

BOWLER'S SWING
(hold that tummy in)

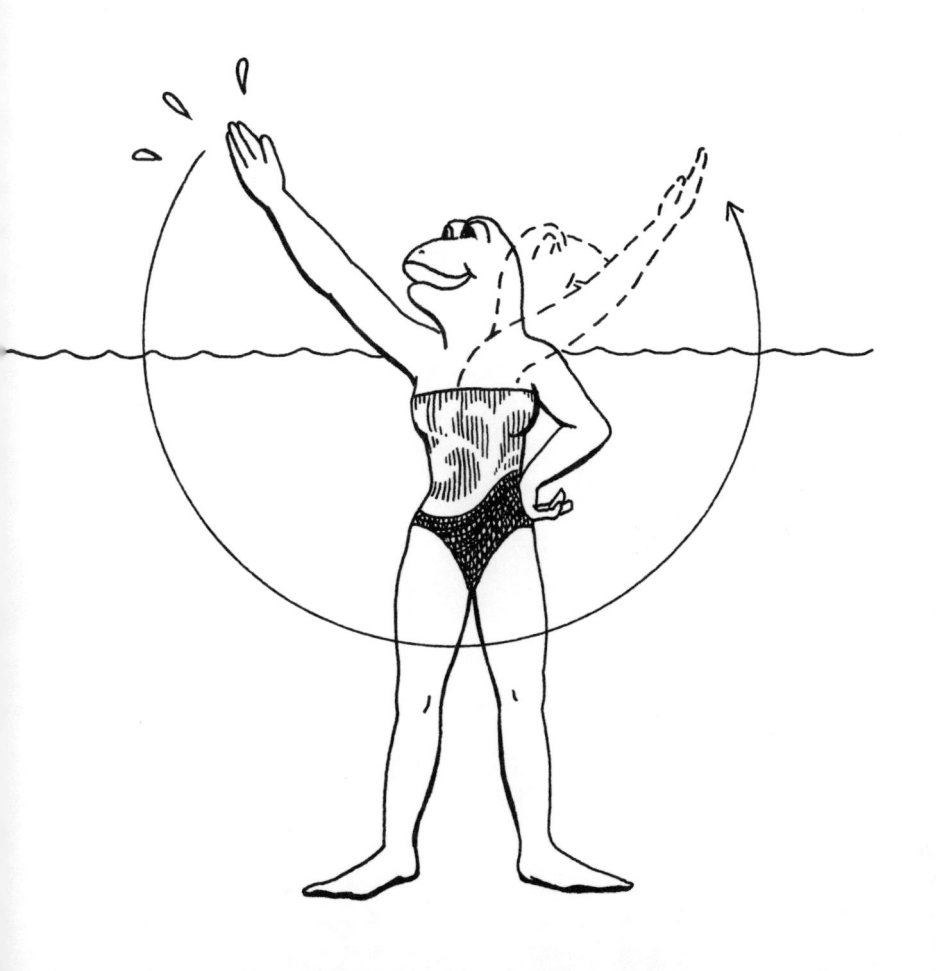

GOLFER'S SWING

Jug, n. 1. An empty plastic gallon or half gallon container, e.g. a milk, juice or water container. 2. An inexpensive piece of exercise equipment.

Jugging, v. 1. The use of jugs (gallon or half gallon) to give added resistance for exercises. 2. The use of jugs (gallon) as floatation devices.

How to Prepare Jugs, 1. remove label. 2. wash empty jugs out then tighten lid back on top. 3. If the jug deflates remove the lid and blow it back up. 4. If desired draw pictures on the jug with a waterproof marker.

JUGGING

JUGGING RULES

1. Trust the jugs, they'll hold you up
2. Use a loose grip or a straight hand through the handle
3. Keep shoulders relaxed
4. If the jugs are too difficult to submerge with control use only one jug or smaller jugs
5. Use good posture (bottom tucked, tummy in, shoulders relaxed)
6. No bubbles, control the jugs, don't move them too fast
7. To avoid neck strain when lying on your back, keep your chin down
8. When doing sit-ups keep jugs lower than your shoulders, preferably about hip level
9. Remember to Smile

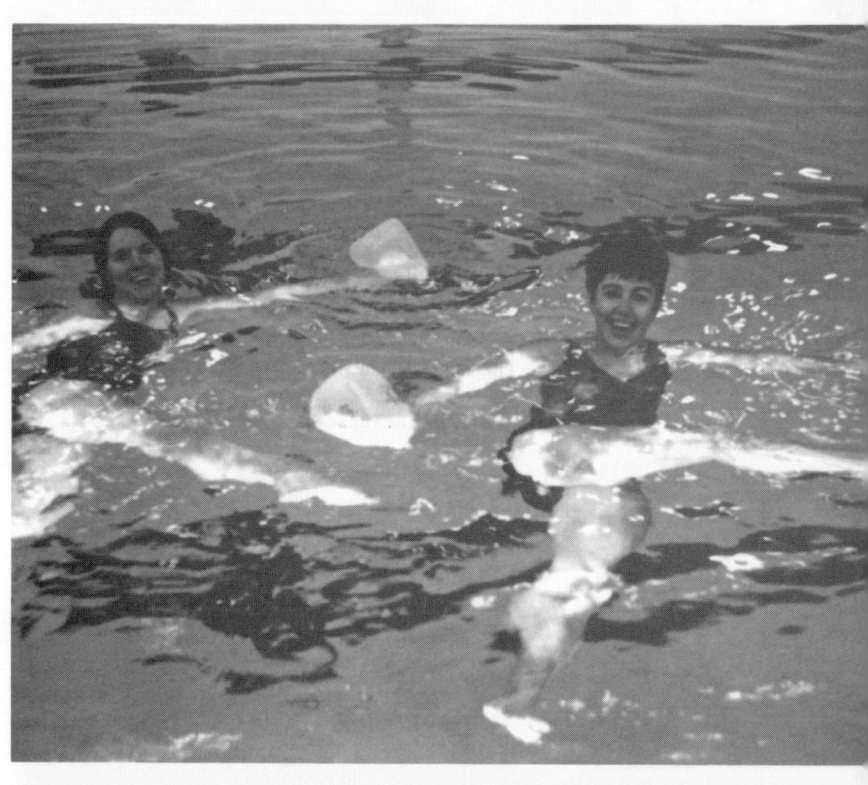

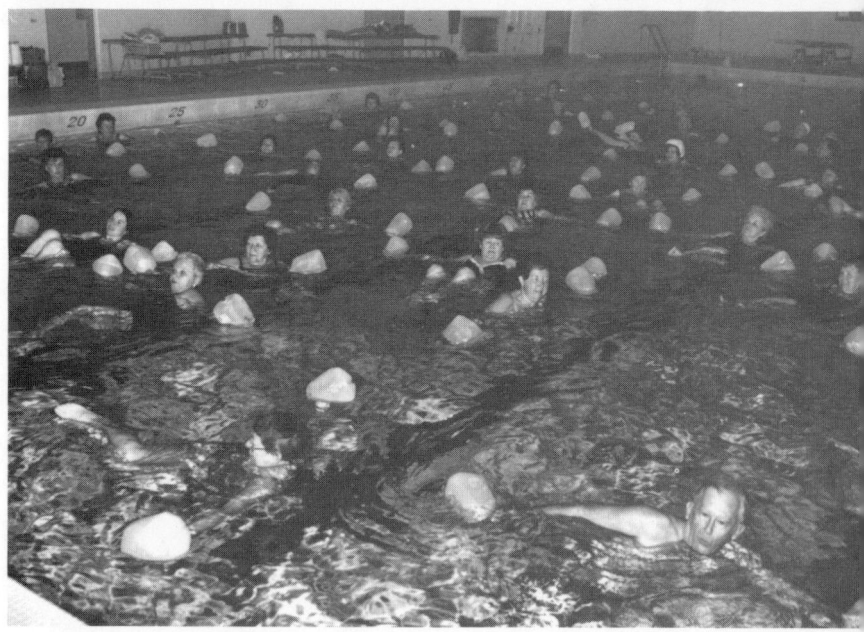

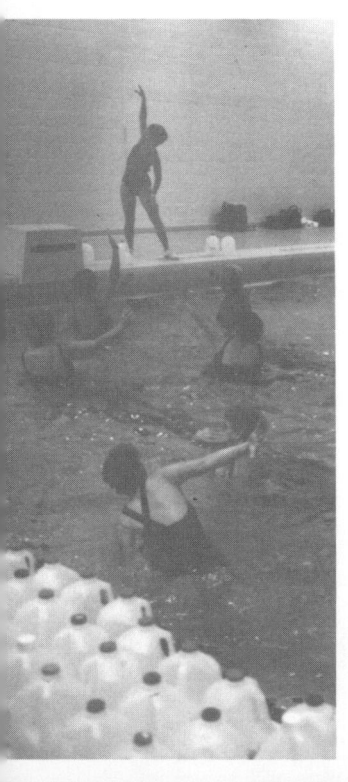

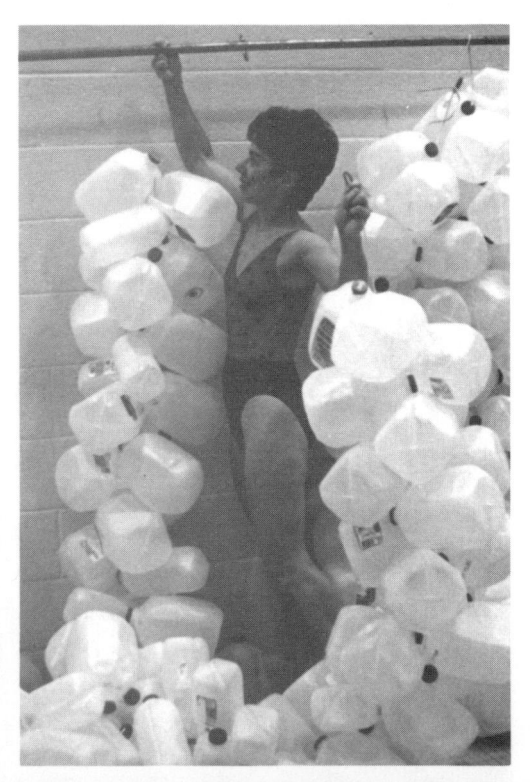

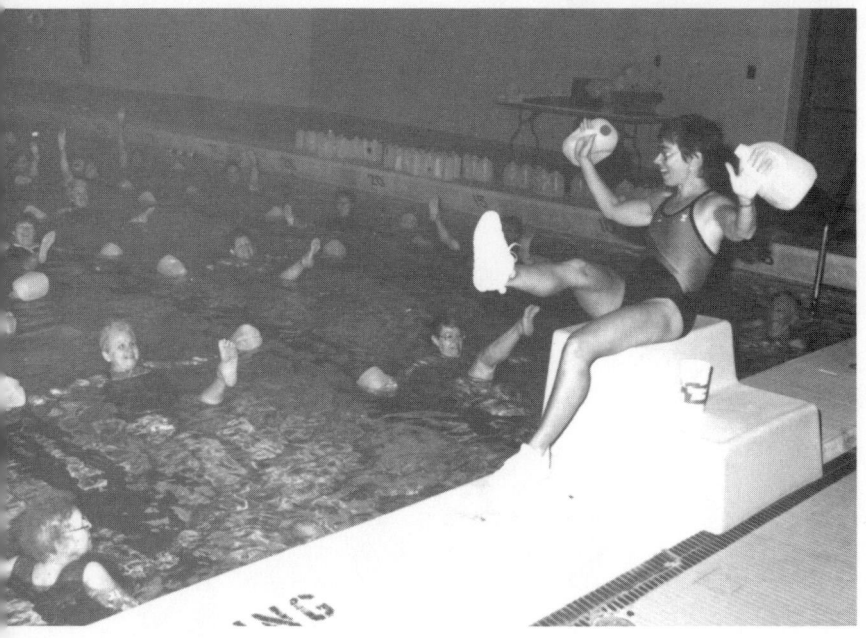

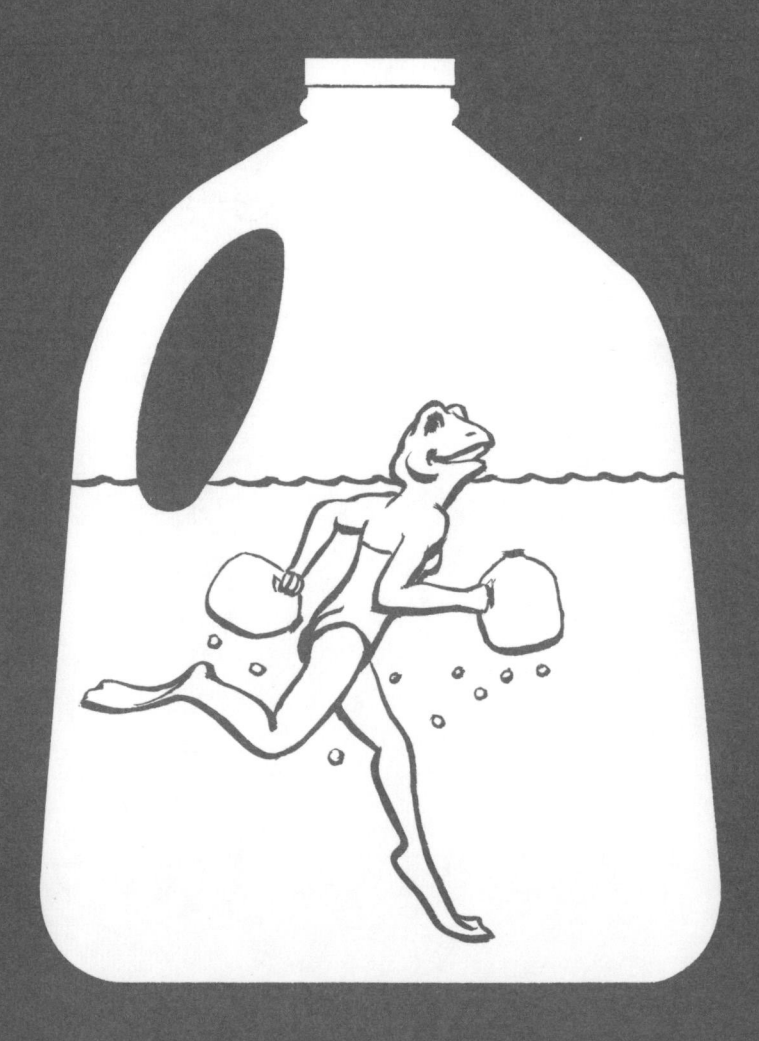

ARMS

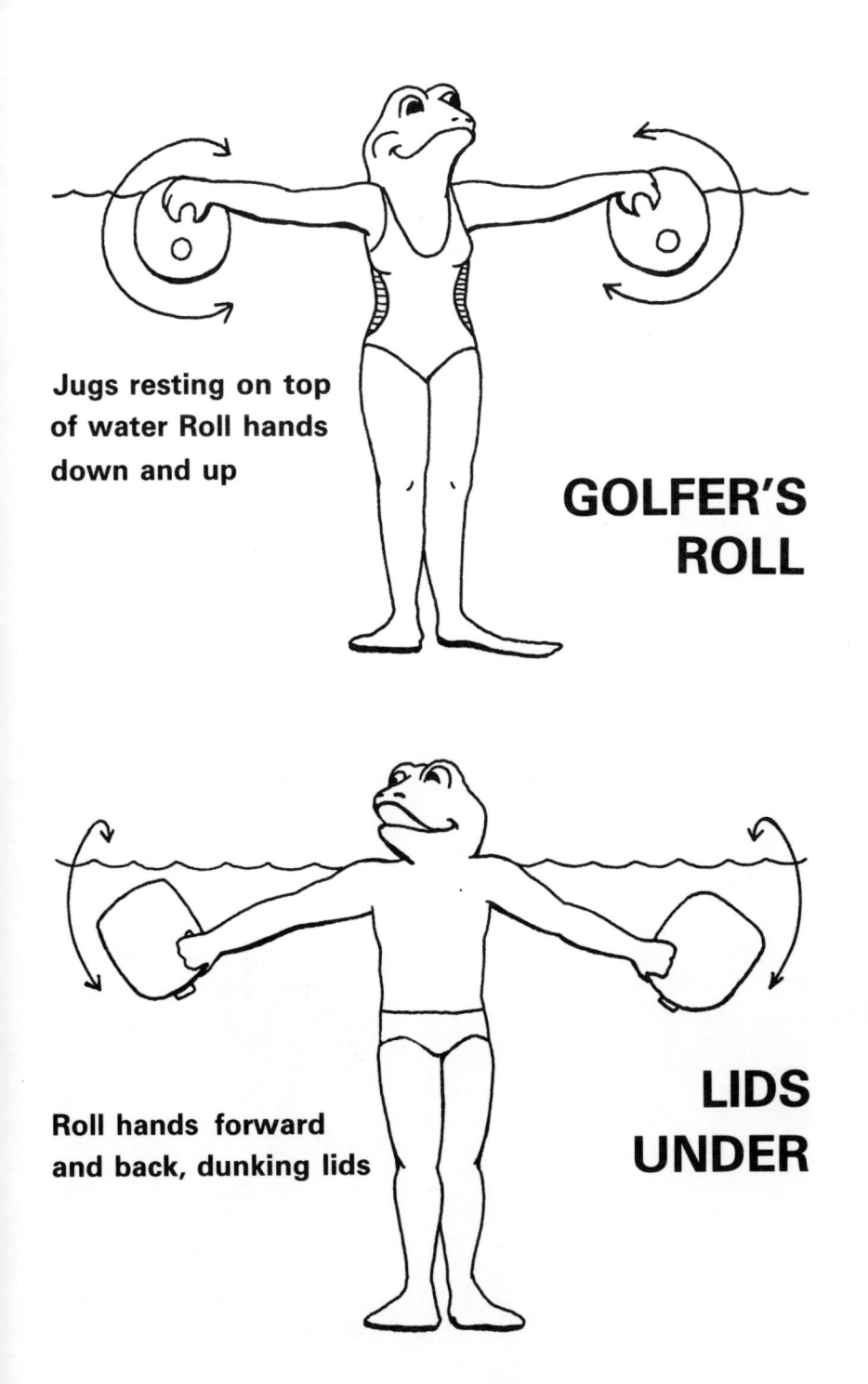

Jugs resting on top of water Roll hands down and up

GOLFER'S ROLL

Roll hands forward and back, dunking lids

LIDS UNDER

JUGGING—ARMS

DOWN AND UPS

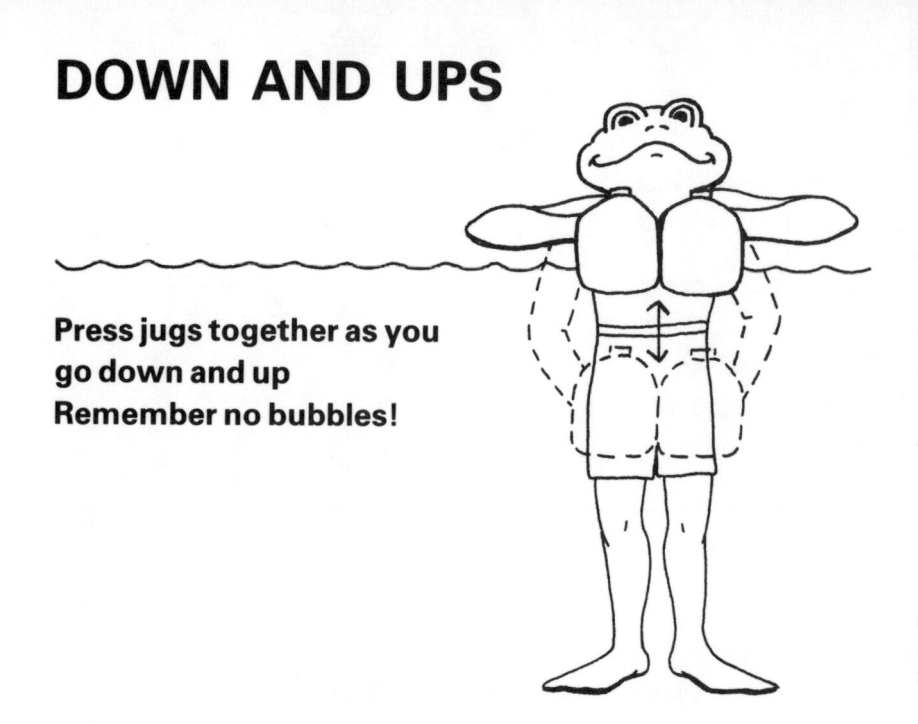

Press jugs together as you
go down and up
Remember no bubbles!

SIDE PULLS

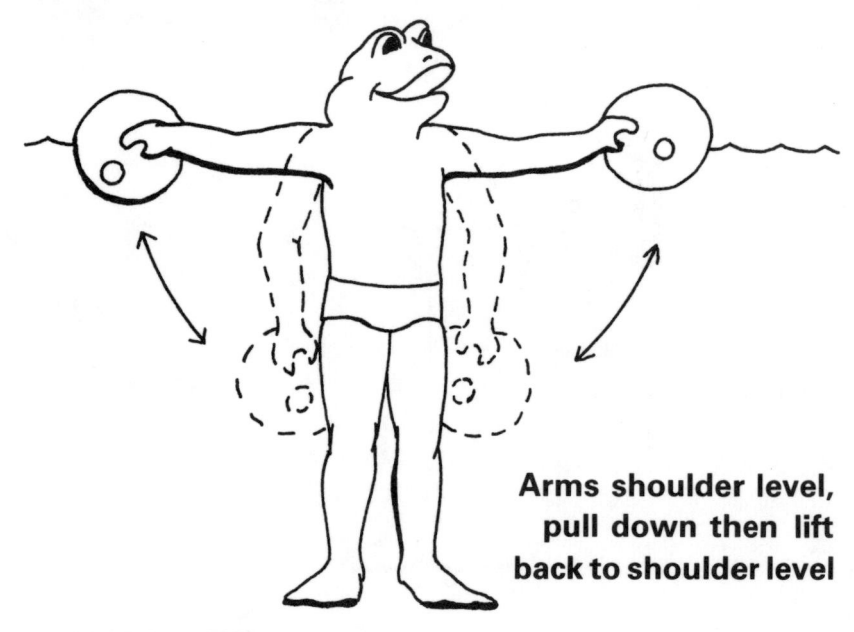

Arms shoulder level,
pull down then lift
back to shoulder level

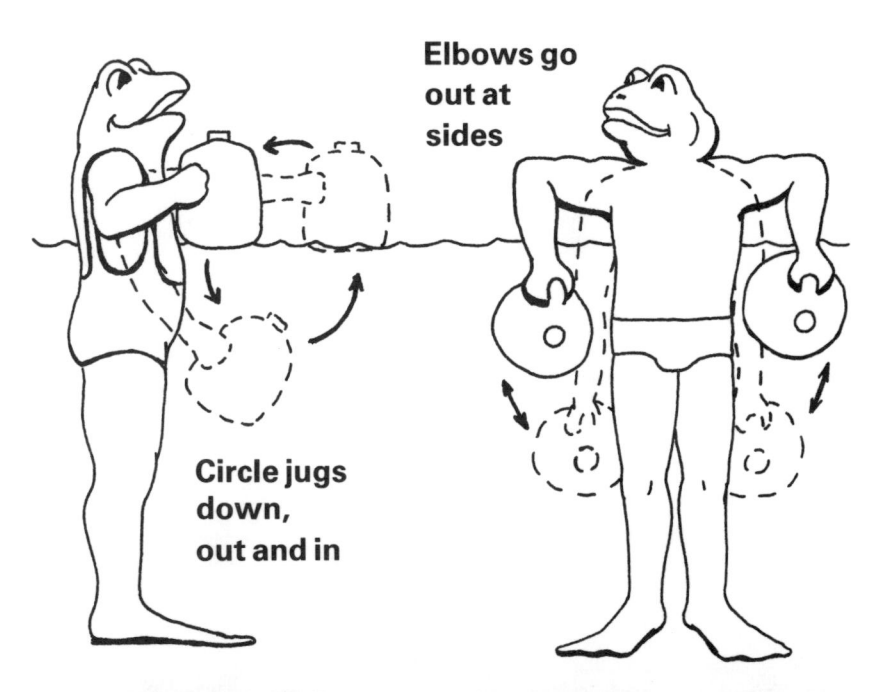

CIRCLES

Circle jugs down, out and in

ELBOW LIFTS

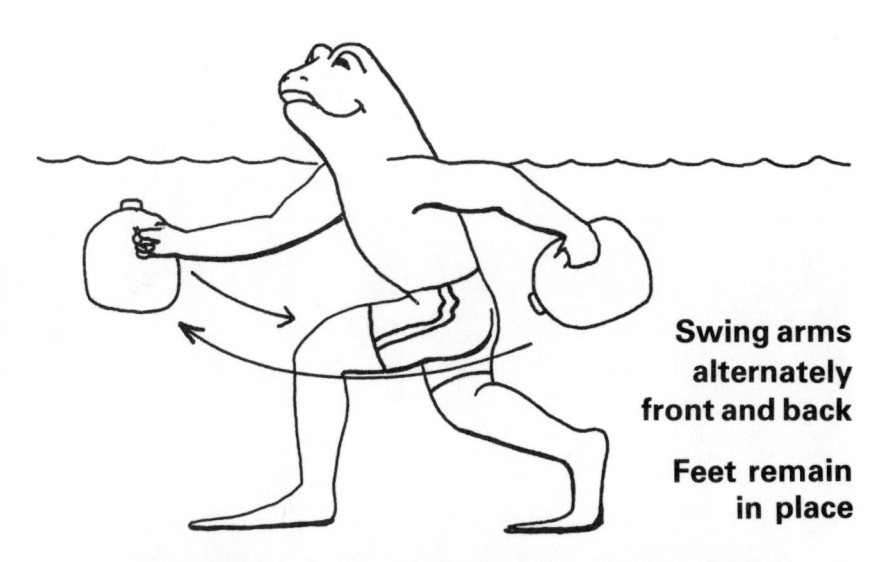

Elbows go out at sides

CROSS COUNTRY SKIING

Swing arms alternately front and back

Feet remain in place

JUGGING—ARMS 85

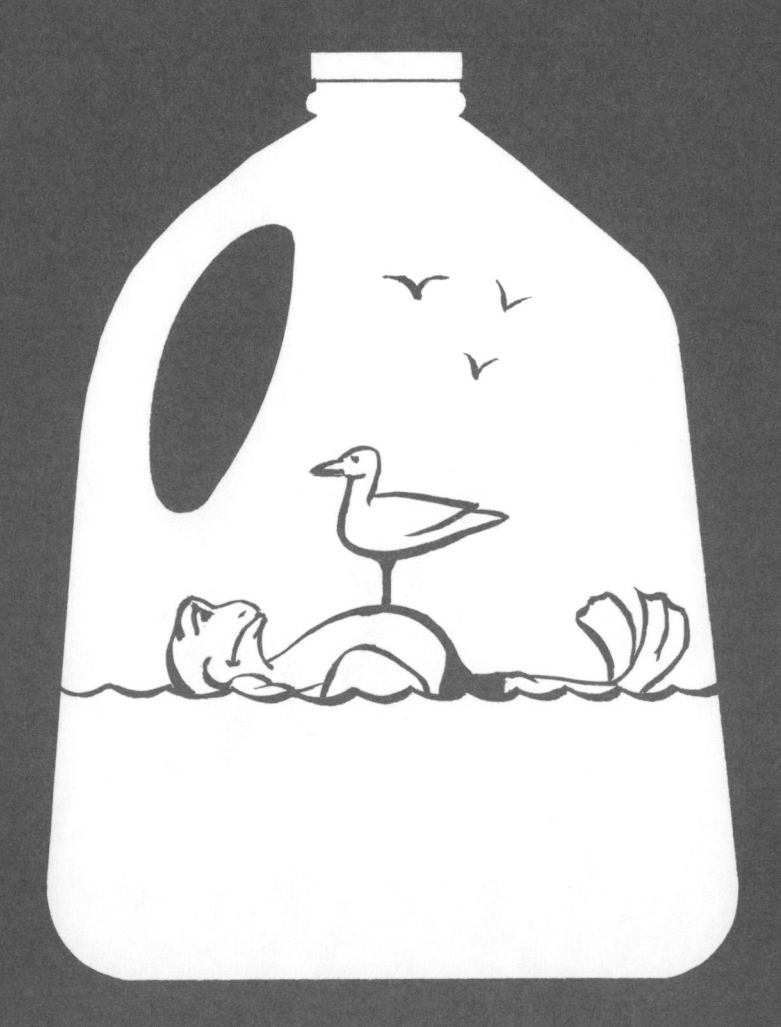

WAIST AND ABDOMEN

"W'S"

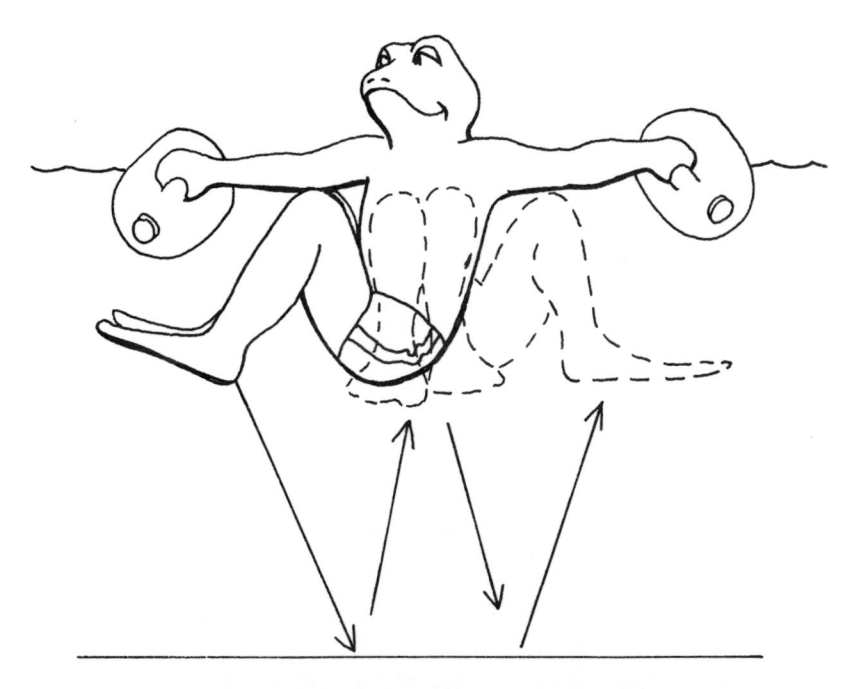

Touch floor before each tuck

HIP ROLLS

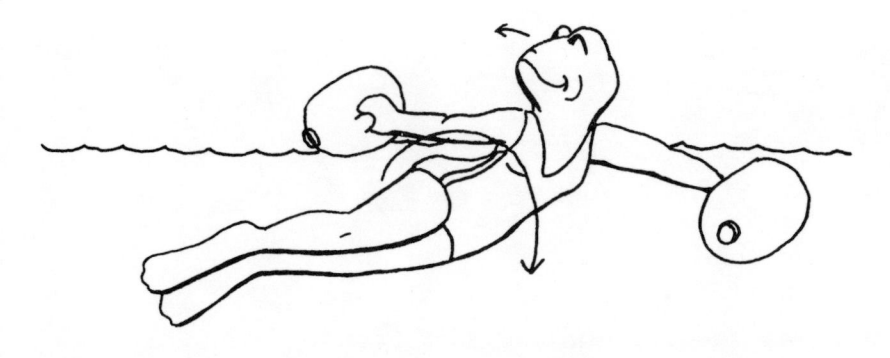

Shoulders remain still Roll hips right and left, look in the opposite direction

JUGGING—WAIST AND ABDOMEN

JUG KICK

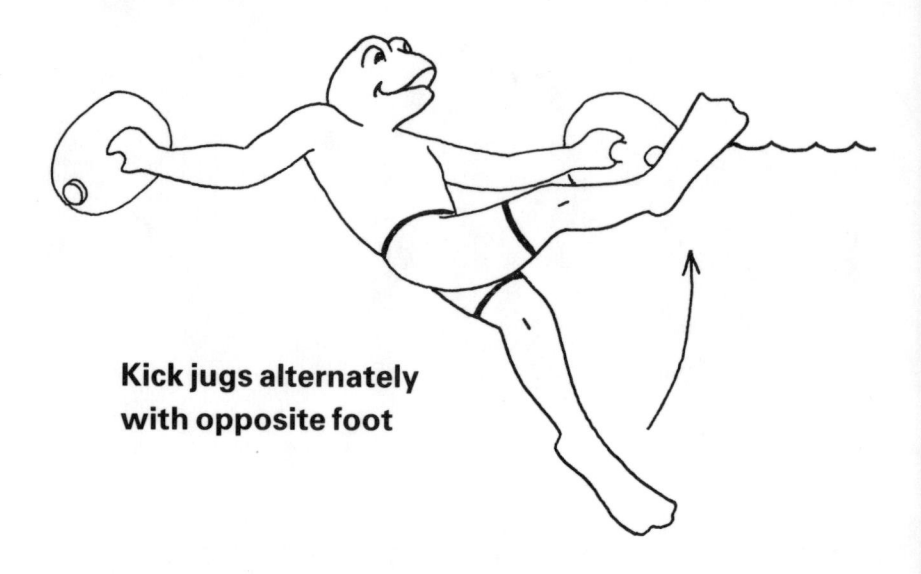

Kick jugs alternately with opposite foot

TUMMY CRUNCH

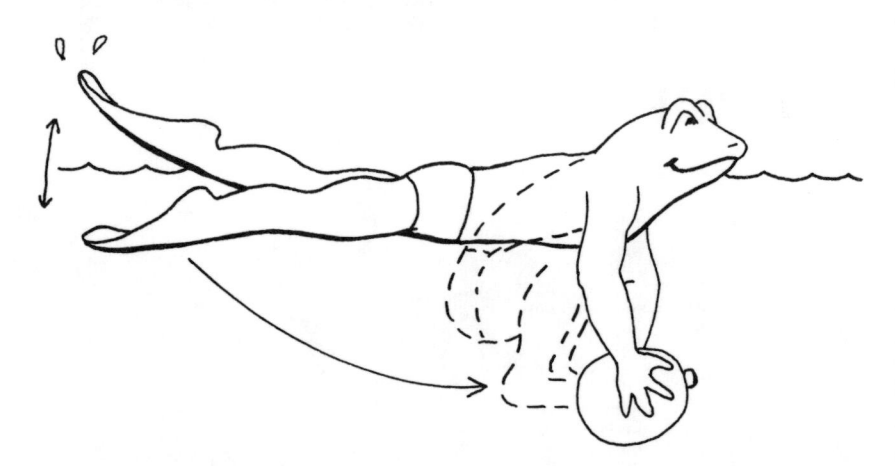

Arms under shoulders, kick 4 times, scrunch to touch toes to jugs then kick again and repeat

BALLET LEGS

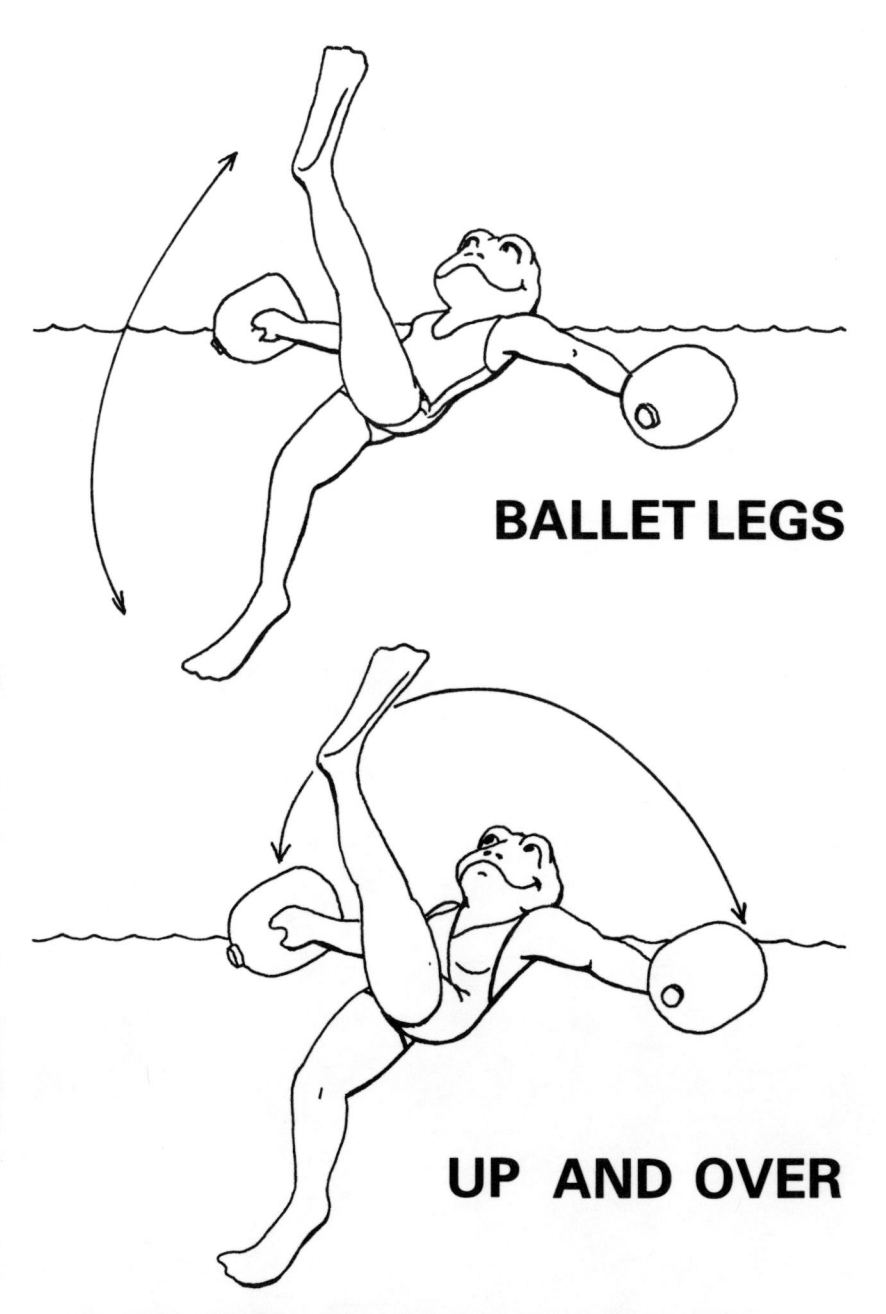

UP AND OVER

Up into a ballet leg, take toe to opposite jug,
straight up then to other jug,
straight up again then slowly come down

FROGGY SWING

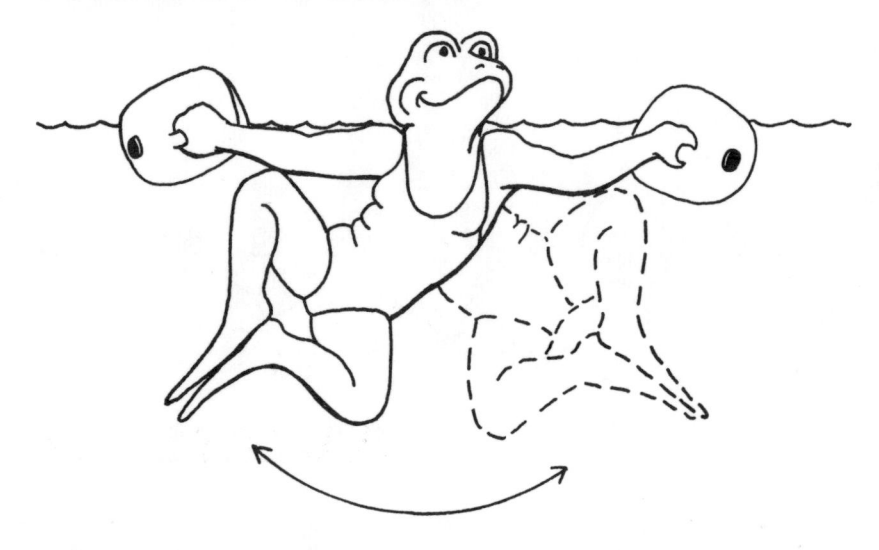

Toes toward floor then swing side to side

FROGGY SWING AND STRETCH

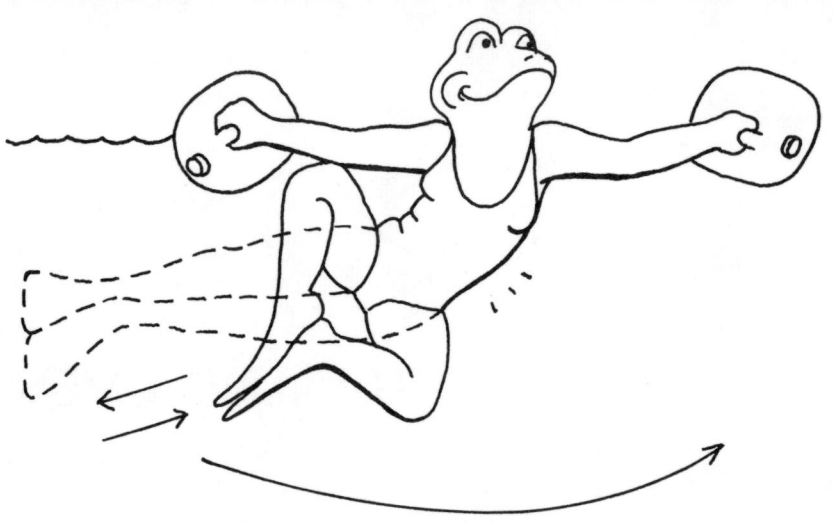

On side swing, stretch legs out to side
then tuck and swing to other side

94 JUGGING—WAIST AND ABDOMEN

JUG TAPS

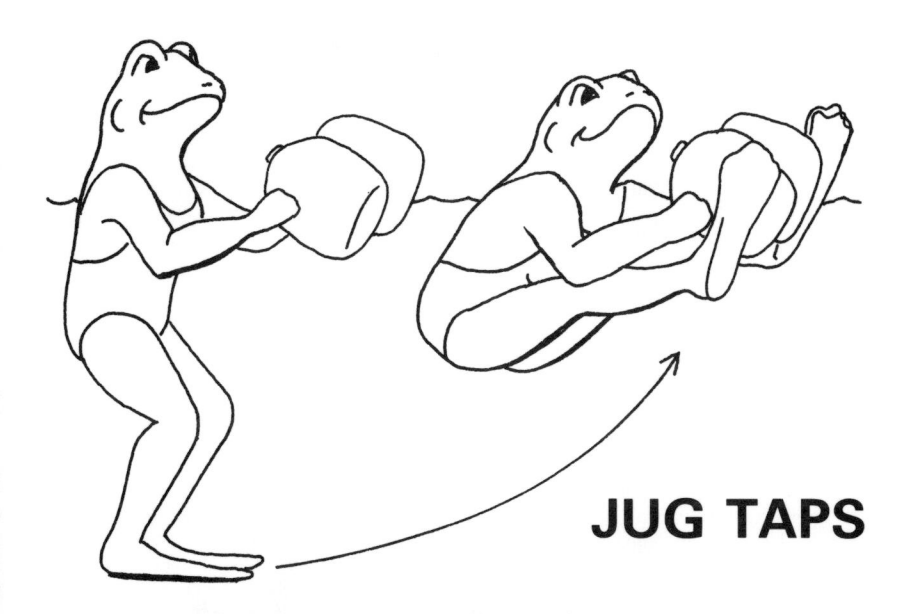

Stand legs apart, knees slightly bent,
jugs slightly forward
Take feet up towards jugs and back to floor

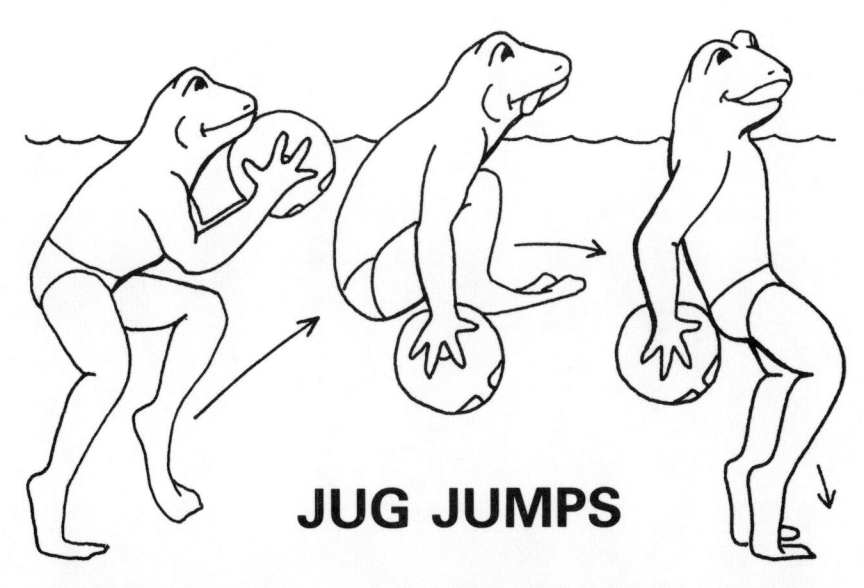

JUG JUMPS

Jog 5 steps Jump over the jug and repeat sequence

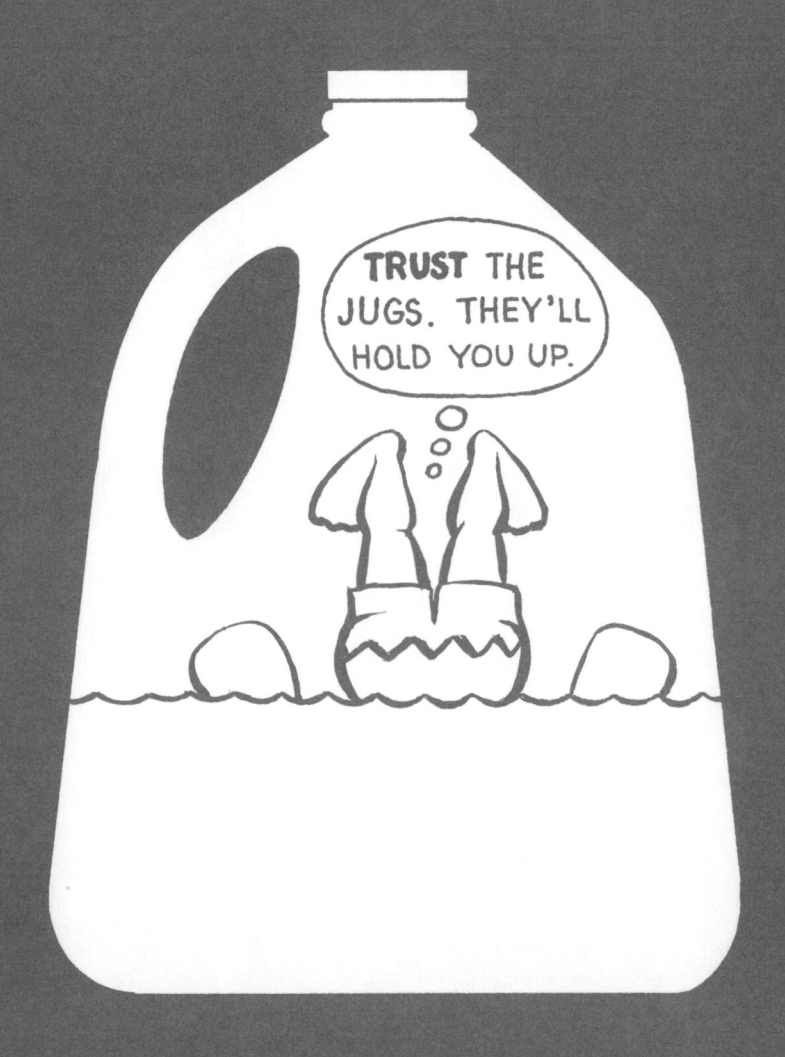

THIGHS AND HIPS

PIGEON TOES

**Sit up tall Back straight Legs straight out in front
Lead with heels out and in**

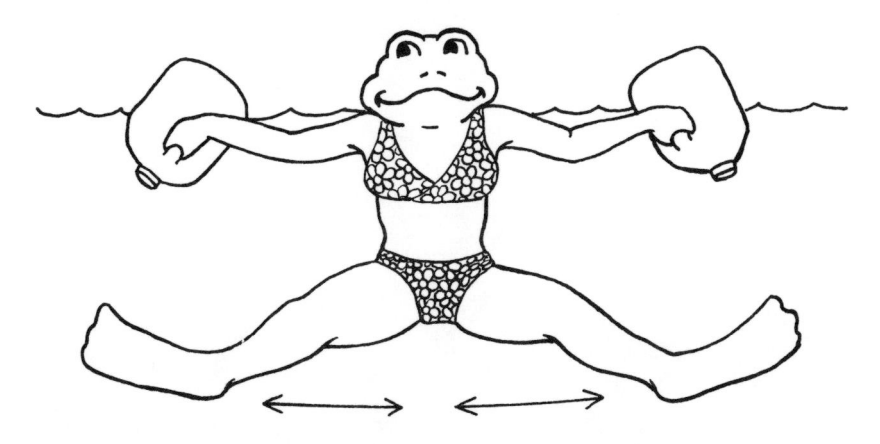

PIGEON PULSES

**Legs wide apart, toes turned in
Do little pulses with toes towards the center**

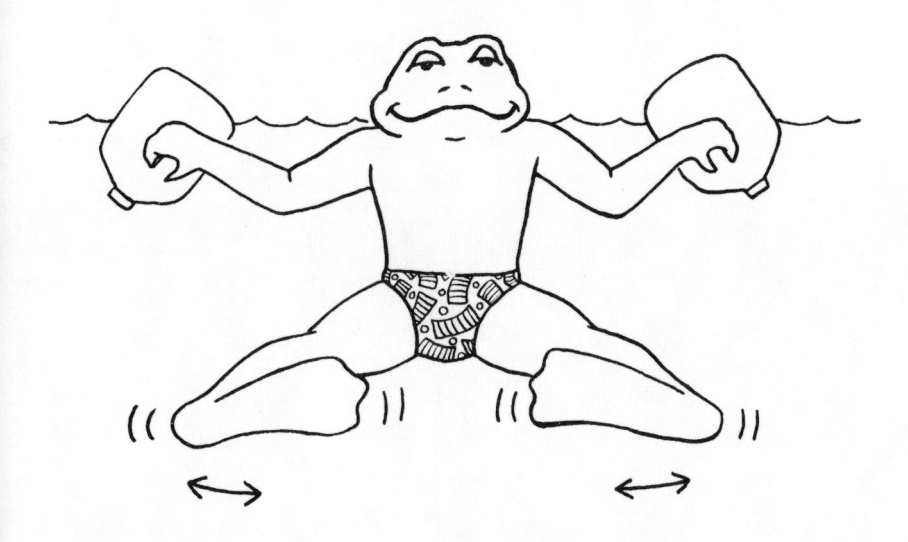

CIRCLES

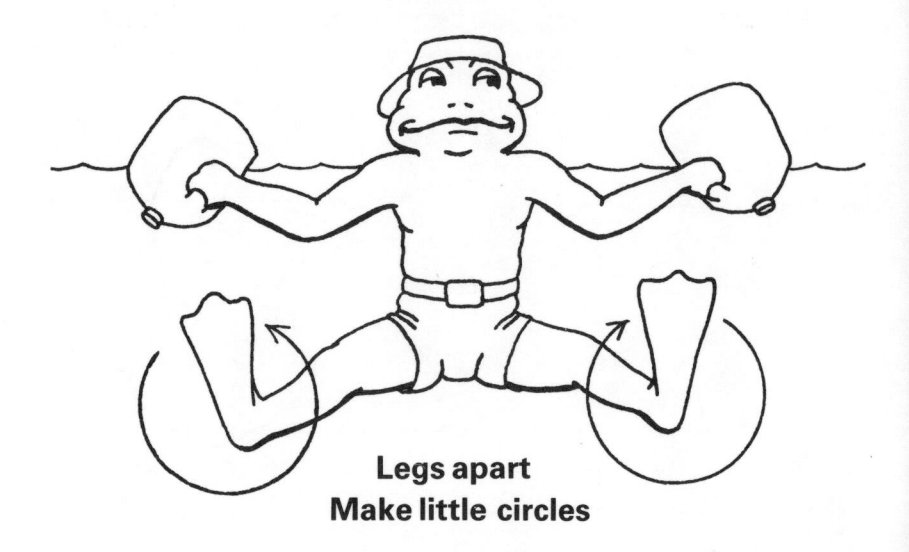

**Legs apart
Make little circles**

FROG LEGS

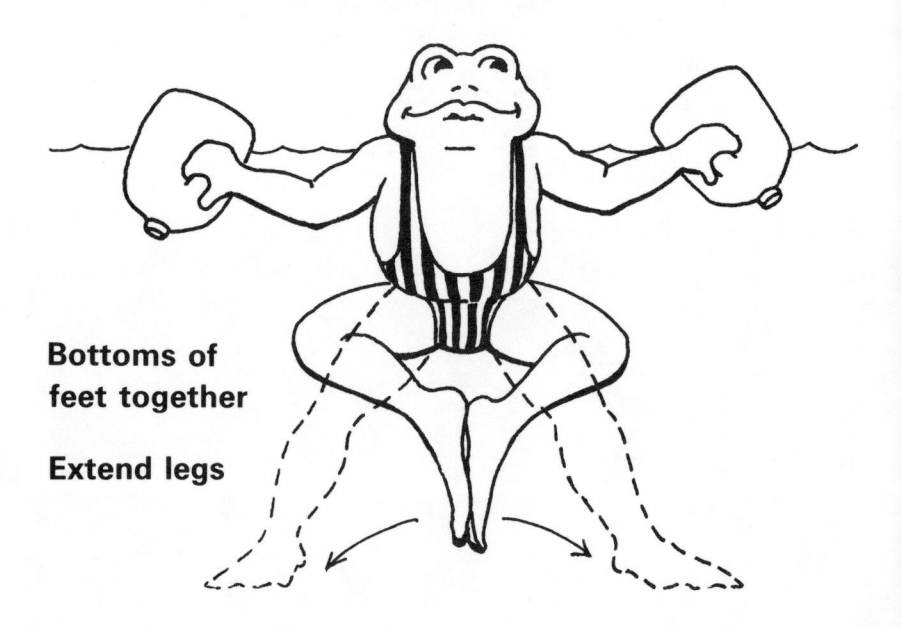

**Bottoms of
feet together**

Extend legs

100 JUGGING—THIGHS AND HIPS

WIDE CRISS-CROSSES

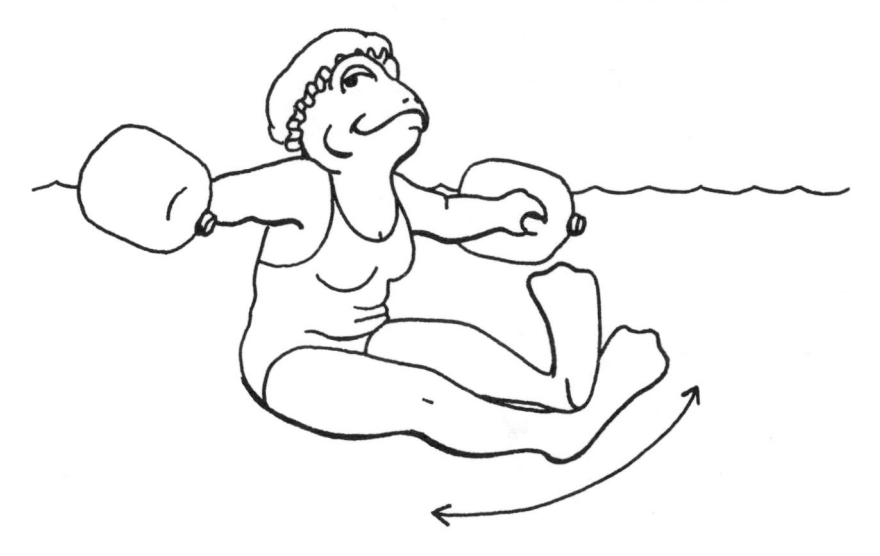

LITTLE CRISS-CROSSES

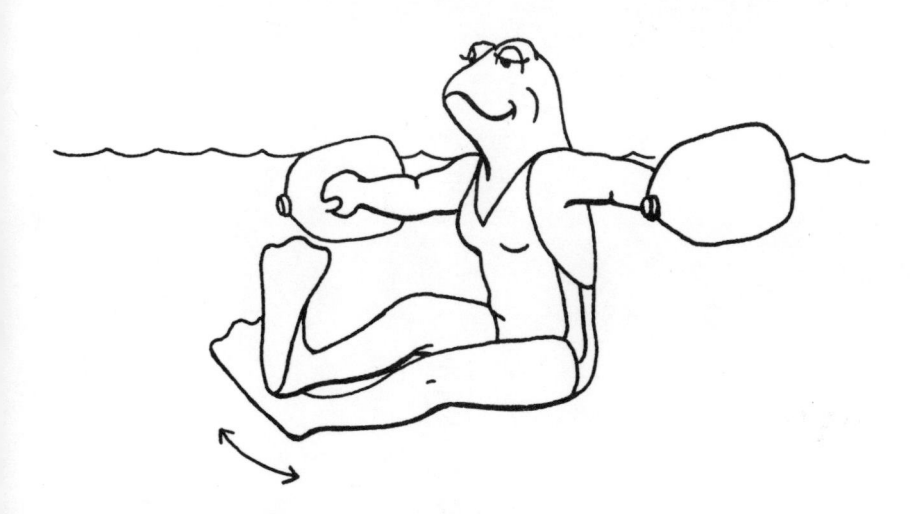

JUGGING—THIGHS AND HIPS

FLOOR TOUCHES

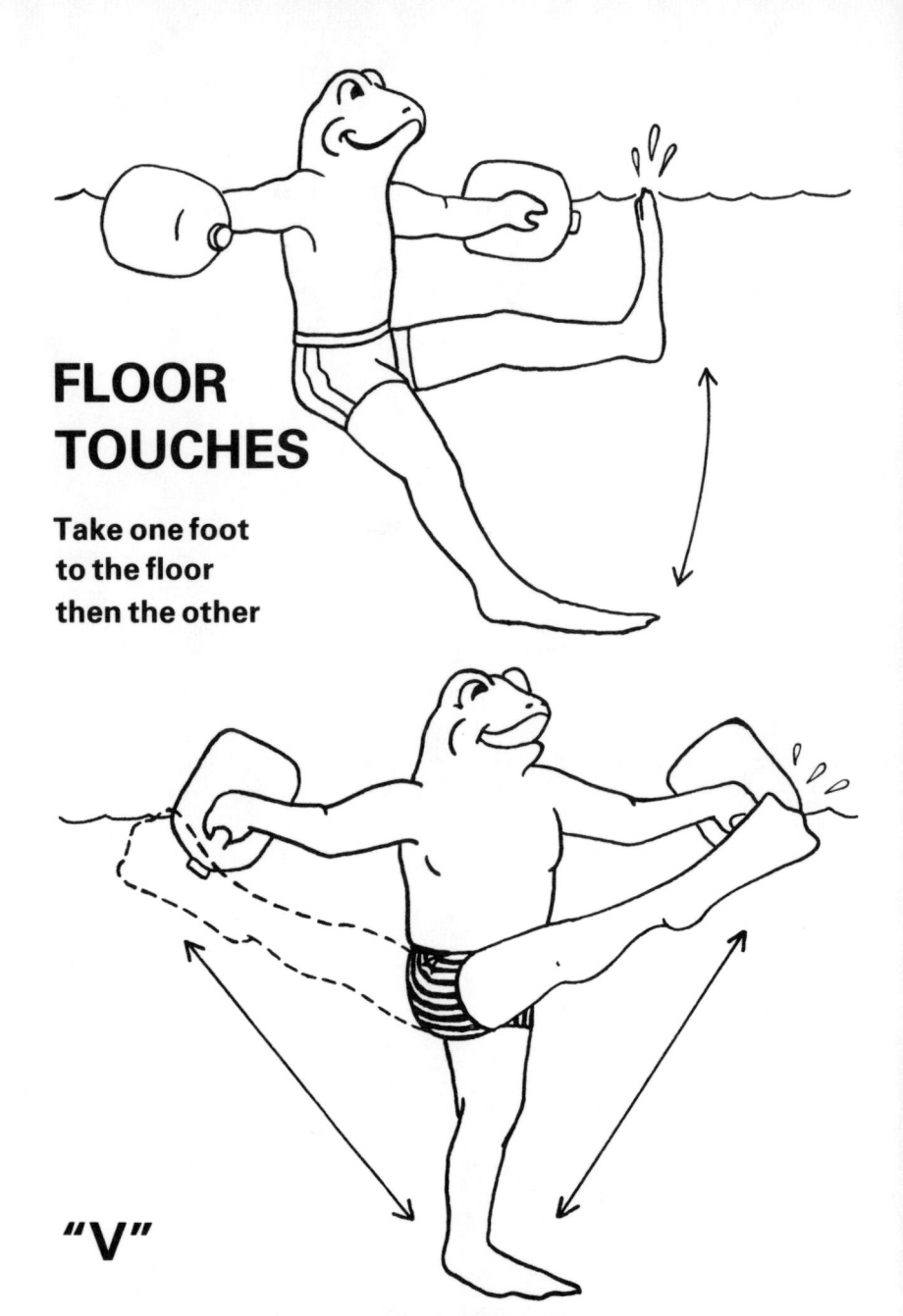

Take one foot to the floor then the other

"V"

Touch foot to alternate jugs forming "V" by touching the floor inbetween
Do 10 with one leg   Repeat with the other leg

MY PROGRESS

DATE:	DATE:
HIPS	HIPS
WAIST	WAIST
BUST/CHEST	BUST/CHEST
R. THIGH	R. THIGH
L. THIGH	L. THIGH
R. UPPER ARM	R. UPPER ARM
L. UPPER ARM	L. UPPER ARM

DATE:	DATE:
HIPS	HIPS
WAIST	WAIST
BUST/CHEST	BUST/CHEST
R. THIGH	R. THIGH
L. THIGH	L. THIGH
R. UPPER ARM	R. UPPER ARM
L. UPPER ARM	L. UPPER ARM

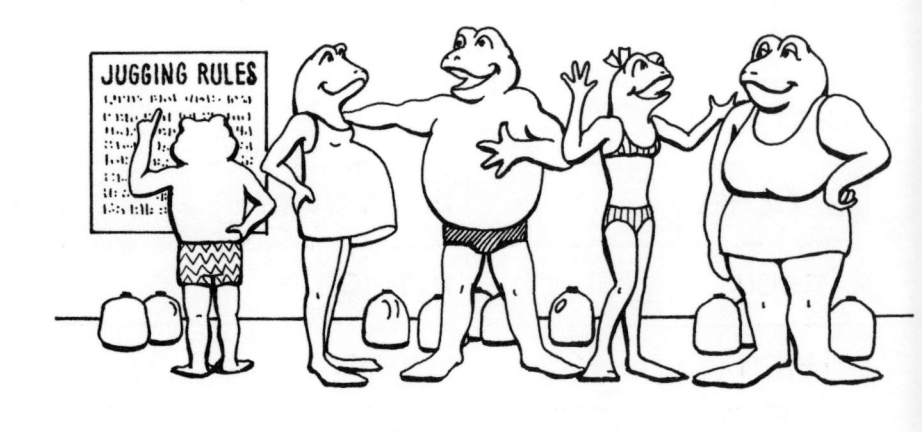

BOOK ORDER FORM

Please send me _____ copies of SHAPE-UP WITH SPLASH @ $10.95 I am enclosing $2.00 for postage and handling. I understand that it will take three weeks for delivery.

Checks payable to: Judy's Splash Aerobics
Michigan residents add 4% sales tax

NAME _____

STREET _____

CITY _____ STATE _____ ZIP _____

CLEANSING CONTENTMENT

I dive into the pool; the cold water shocking my warm body, startling me wide awake. My tensions are jarred from their hiding places. I become aware of tightened shoulders, a clenched jaw, or a pain that throbs up from my neck to pulsate behind an eye. Each morning when I come to this cleansing place, I bring yesterday's burdens with me.

I join others and we get right to work; first traveling continuously back and forth across the pool; jogging, striding, leaping, hopping. Then we float, we flip, we curl up and stretch. We are seals, dogs, fishes, frogs, as we go through awkward, yet graceful, movements.

We target parts of our bodies; twisting to trim the waist, jumping to tighten the abdomen, pulling to firm the arms, kicking to strengthen the legs. Heart rates increase, pumping blood through arteries to oxygen-starved extremities; pushing the worries and tensions ever nearer to the surface.

Then, as the activity slows down, water which has surrounded the body, continuously massaging the skin, releases the tenseness, which floats away; leaving a feeling of warmth, relaxation, and delicious contentment. We have cleansed ourselves of yesterday's burdens and now are ready to begin a new day.

Joyce Callow Motta

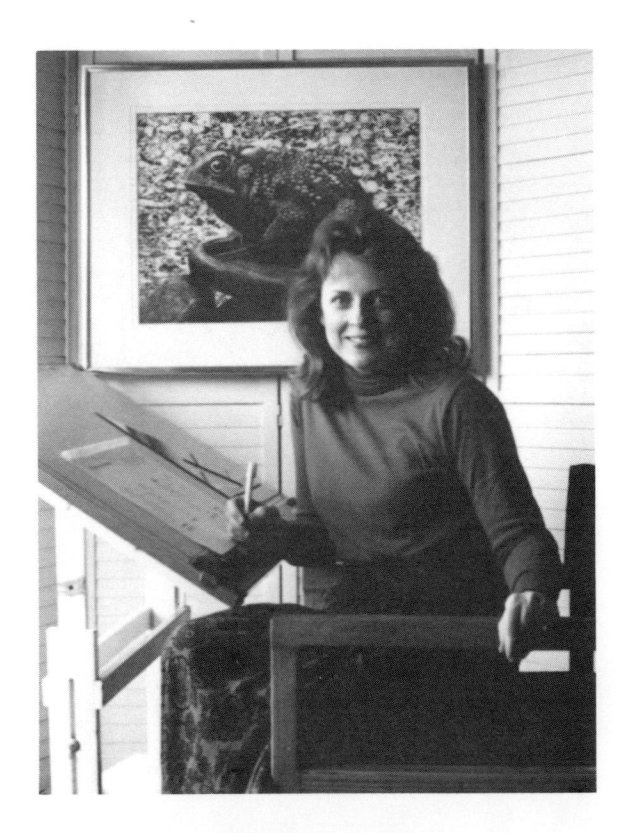

ILLUSTRATOR

C. Gundy Guskey has studied art at the University of Pittsburgh, Columbus College of Art and Design, Michigan State University and the Allgemeine Gewerbeschule Basel. Her commissioned works hang in England, Switzerland, Germany and throughout the United States.

Research for this book was done while attending three months of the author's *Splash Aerobics* classes. During this time the water exercises, coupled with a change in diet, helped Gundy lose considerable weight and inches, while greatly increasing her energy level.

A love of water (but not exercise) and a lifelong fascination with frogs, toads and human nature has combined to create the new species of "everyday athletes" in this book. Any resemblance of them to her water exercise classmates should be taken with a grain of salt!

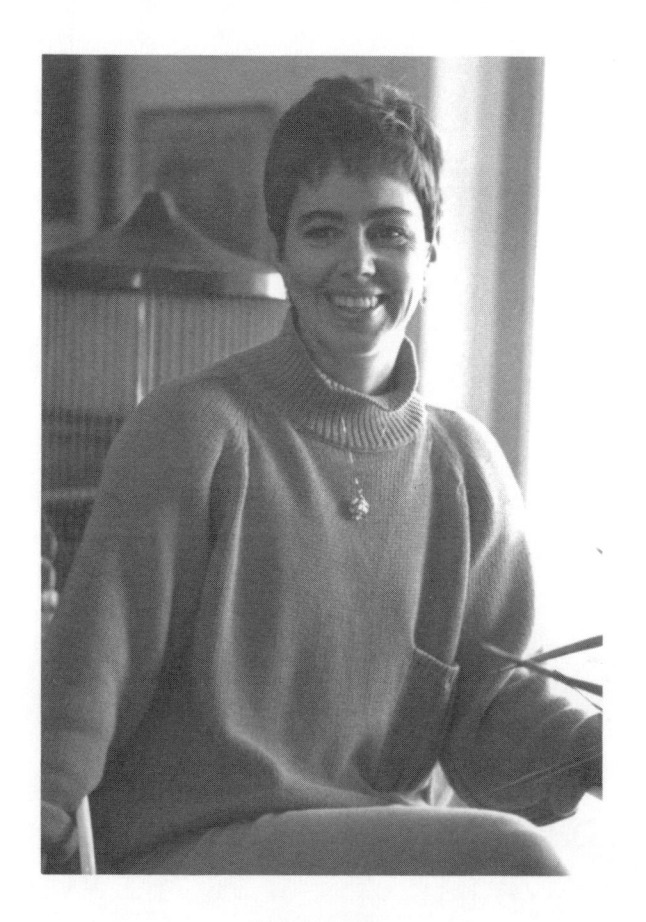

AUTHOR

Judy Davenport Conley earned a degree in Physical Education from Arizona State University. She has many years of experience teaching swimming, fitness and aerobic classes to all ages.

In addition to running her rapidly growing company, *Judy's Splash Aerobics*, she is an instructor in the Athletic Department of Lansing Community College. Judy's expertise is recognized by the Arthritis Foundation and she is certified to teach their Aquatic Arthritis program.

Being an active volunteer in her church and community as well as the proud mother of eight children, Judy brings enthusiasm and infectious energy to everything she does.

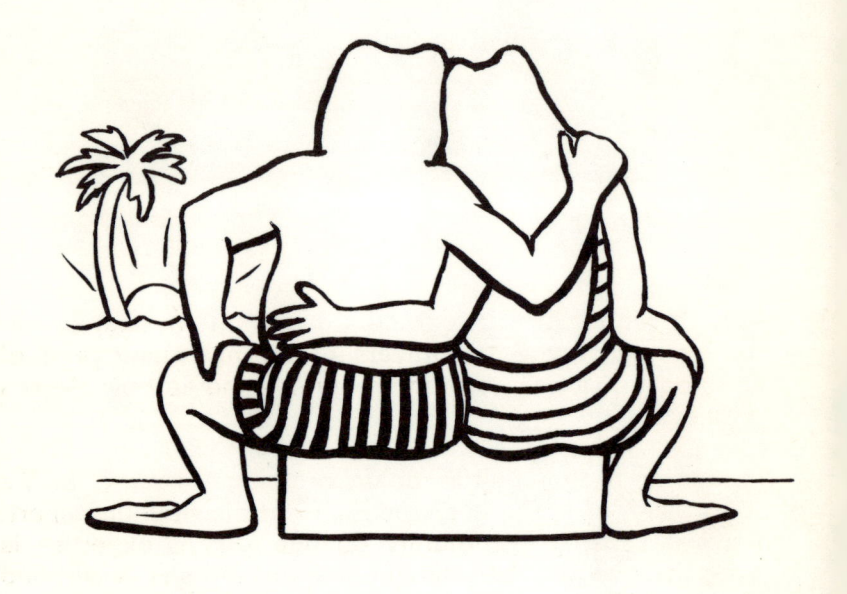

More Sites to Surf

If you just can't get enough insect stuff, a visit to these sites will keep you buzzing!

Take a virtual tour of the O. Orkin Insect Zoo!
http://www.orkin.com/html/insect_zoo.html

See movies and closeups of your favorite insects!
http://www.ent.iastate.edu/imagegallery/

Visit the Antlion Pit for a look at the doodlebug!
http://www.actionpit.com

Check out the wonderful world of insects!
http://www.earthlife.net/insects/six.html

Explore a ton of insect links!
http://www.neartica.com/family/kids/kbugs.htm

Photo Credits

Charles Abramson p7; **David G. Campbell/Visuals Unlimited** p17; **Corel** p2, p4, p5, p6, p8, p11, p12, p15, p17, p18, p19, p20, p21, p22, p23; **David M. Dennis/Tom Stack** p4, p7, p10, p11; **Mark Griffiths** p15; **Ken Lucas/Visuals Limited** p14; **RCMP** p5; **John Shaw** p12; **Tom Stack** p9; **J.D. Taylor:** p13; **Joyce Wang** p16

Are spiders a type of insect?

finditquick @ http://www.letsfindout.com/subjects/bug/rfispsta.html

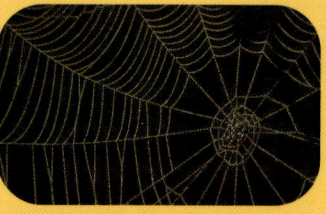

Daddy Many Legs

Spiders are related to insects, but the two are different in many ways. All spiders have eight legs, while insects have only six. Most insects have wings and antennae, but spiders have neither. A spider's body is divided into two parts, while an insect's body is divided into three parts.

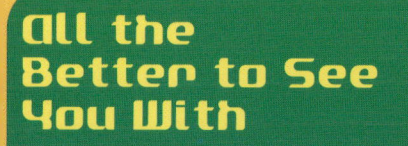

All the Better to See You With

Most insects have two large compound eyes and, sometimes, other simple eyes. Spiders usually have eight simple eyes.

Itsy, Bitsy Spider

The smallest spider in the world is about the size of a period. The largest has a leg span as wide as your computer screen.

Brainteaser

Q What word means a fear of spiders?

A Arachnophobia is a fear of spiders. Insectophobia or entomophobia is a fear of insects.

Which types of fabric do insects make?

finditquick @ http://www.jspca.org.za/antics/silk.html

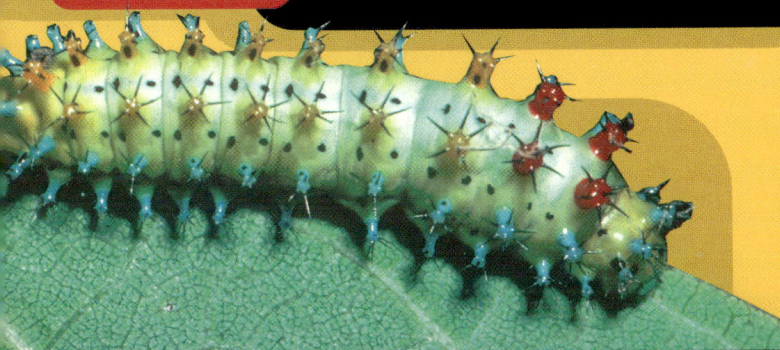

Not a Worm at All

Silkworms are not really worms, but insects in their caterpillar stage. Silkworms create their cocoons out of a fine substance that is woven together to create silk. In three days, one silkworm can create more than 1,800 feet of thread!

Silk Spies

For thousands of years, the silkworm was the secret pride of the Chinese. Other countries sent spies to try to steal the secret of silk making. As silkworm eggs were smuggled out of the country, the silk industry spread throughout the world. One of the most famous trade routes of all time was known as the Silk Road, which carried silk cloth from China to Rome.

Places To Go!

Find out more about the whole silk process—from worms to weaving!

finditquick @

http://www.comptons.com/encyclopedia/ARTICLES/0150/01679616_A.html

Which insect was considered sacred in ancient Egypt?

finditquick @ http://www.letsfindout.com/subjects/bug/rfisacrd.html

Holy Insect!

The scarab beetle is a type of dung-eating beetle. In ancient Egypt, the scarab was considered to be a holy animal. Because of its round shape and golden colors, the scarab represented the sun. The Egyptians believed that Ra, their sun god, sometimes appeared as a scarab.

Beetle Jewelry

The people of ancient Egypt often carved precious stones into the shape of scarab beetles. These beads were worn to bring good luck and to ward off evil. Scarabs are also seen in many Egyptian monuments.

The Immortal Insect

Egyptians and other ancient cultures believed that beetles were symbols of immortality. They thought beetles disappeared into the ground and returned to life when they reappeared.

Things To Do!

Send an insect e-postcard to a fellow insectophile!

finditquick @ http://postcards.www.media.mit.edu/PObin/readRack.perl?Insects.list|Insect+Drawings/

What are the four stages in the life of a butterfly?

finditquick @ http://www1.bos.nl/homes/bijlmakers/entomology/begin.htm

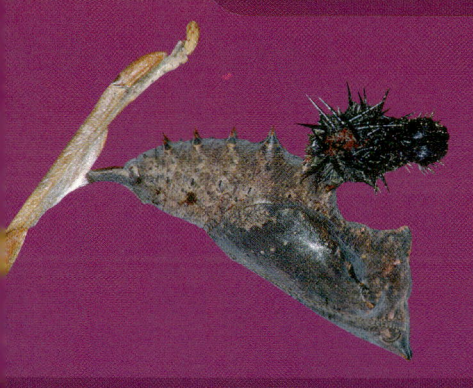

Cozy Cocoons

Butterflies don't start out beautiful—they have to go through something called metamorphosis. They begin their lives as eggs, which hatch into larvae, or caterpillars. The larvae spin cocoons and turn into pupae. Adult butterflies and moths then emerge from these cocoons.

The Simple Life

Some insects go through incomplete metamorphosis, which consists of three stages instead of four. These insects do not have a pupal stage. Instead, they begin their lives as eggs, which hatch into larvae. The insects' wings grow during the larval stage. The larvae look very similar to the adult insects, only smaller. The larvae shed several layers of skin and grow until they become adults.

Brainteaser

Q How much water does a moth drink?

A Pound for pound, a human would have to drink one gallon per second to keep up with a moth.

Why do bees make honey?

finditquick @ http://www.honey.com/kids/facts.html

Fit for a Queen

Bees collect juice, or nectar, from flowers and bring it back to the hive to feed the queen bee and the larvae. Bees make honey to eat during the winter when plants are not flowering and producing nectar.

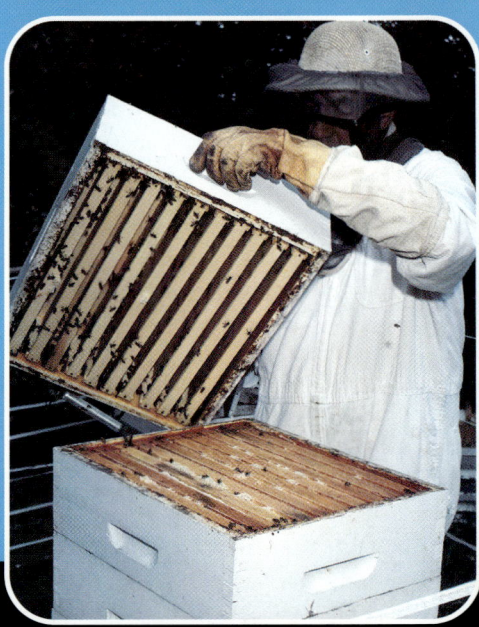

Leftovers

The European honeybee, which is found in North America, makes huge amounts of honey--much more than the bees in the hive could ever eat. Because of this, people can remove honey from the hives for humans to use.

Honey, I'm Home

Worker bees are all females who are unable to mate or lay eggs. Worker bees collect nectar and make honey. Workers feed the queen, take care of the young larvae, and guard the entrance to the hive.

Places To Go!

See the world through the eyes of a bee!

finditquick @

http://cvs.anu.edu.au/andy/beye/beyehome.html

What do you call someone who studies insects?

finditquick @ http://www.entsoc.org/education/what_is.html

Bug Work

Do insects fascinate you? You may want to become an entomologist—someone who studies insects. Some people study insects as a hobby, while others work as professional entomologists.

Creature Comforts

Entomologists study how insects spread disease and try to learn how to prevent them from attacking crops. They also learn about useful insects, like the honeybee, which can be helpful to people, plants, and animals. The Entomological Society of America is an organization for people interested in studying insects.

An Ancient Science

People have been examining and using insects for thousands of years. The philosopher Aristotle studied insects in ancient Greece. The Chinese first began making silk with silkworms in 4700 BCE.

Things To Do!

Model your favorite insect in *papier-maché*.

finditquick @ http://www.uky.edu/Agriculture/Entomology/ythfacts/bugfun/papermch.htm

When do ladybugs play "dead"?

finditquick @ http://insected.arl.arizona.edu/ladyinfo.htm

Playing Defense

When ladybugs are threatened, they will fall to the ground and play dead. Ladybugs can also secrete a bad-tasting liquid, which makes them less attractive as a meal to birds and other predators.

The Early Years

Female ladybugs lay clusters of yellow eggs on leaves. When the eggs hatch, the emerging larvae are wingless and will shed their skin to become pupae. When the adult ladybug finally breaks free, it must wait for its wings to harden before it can fly.

An Appetite for Aphids

A favorite food of adult ladybugs is the aphid, a tiny, flying insect. Ladybugs also eat other small insects, such as scales and mites. Ladybugs prefer to live on plants rich with aphids, like roses and broccoli.

Brainteaser

Q What color are head lice?

A Head lice are clear when they're born and turn reddish-brown when they start to feed.